STOP DIETING
START LIVING

*5 Foundations for Your Health to
Permanently Lose Weight Without
Dieting, Starvation or Suffering in Silence*

ELLIE SAVOY

DFH PRESS
NEW YORK

STOP DIETING START LIVING

5 Foundations for Your Health to Permanently Lose Weight Without Dieting, Starvation or Suffering in Silence

by ELLIE SAVOY

ISBN 978-0-9861042-6-8

Manufactured in the United States of America

Published by:

DFH PRESS
P.O. Box 595
Millbrook, New York 12545
www.DietFreeAndHealthy.com

Interior and Cover Design by:
Rory Carruthers
www.RoryCarruthers.com

For more information about Ellie Savoy or to book her for your next event or media interview please visit: www.DietFreeAndHealthy.com

This book is dedicated to all the women of this world
who want to live a fun, delicious life free of diets,
rules, deprivation and restrictions.

To

Scott & Chris,

Abvndant Health
and Happiness,

Ellie

To Scott & Chris,

Abundant Health
and Happiness.

Ellie

CONTENTS

Introduction _ 1
PART ONE: PRIORITIES _ _ _ _ _ _ _ _ _ _ _ _ _ _ _ _ 7
Are You Missing From Your Life? _ _ _ _ _ _ _ _ _ _ _ _ 9
There Will Never Be the "Perfect" Time _ _ _ _ _ _ _ _ 21
Re-Evaluating What Is Important In Life _ _ _ _ _ _ _ 29
Having Awareness Of Your Choices _ _ _ _ _ _ _ _ _ 33
PART TWO: PRETENDING _ _ _ _ _ _ _ _ _ _ _ _ _ 37
What's Really Weighing You Down? _ _ _ _ _ _ _ _ _ 39
What Are You Really Hungry For? _ _ _ _ _ _ _ _ _ 47
Why Diets Don't Work _ _ _ _ _ _ _ _ _ _ _ _ _ _ _ _ 51
PART THREE: PERCEPTION _ _ _ _ _ _ _ _ _ _ _ 55
Change Your Perception and Change Your Life _ _ _ _ _ 57
Gifts Come In Many Forms _ _ _ _ _ _ _ _ _ _ _ _ _ 64
Integration, Not Separation _ _ _ _ _ _ _ _ _ _ _ _ _ 69
Investment or Expense? _ _ _ _ _ _ _ _ _ _ _ _ _ _ _ 73
PART FOUR: PLAN _ _ _ _ _ _ _ _ _ _ _ _ _ _ _ _ 77
Progression, Not Perfection! _ _ _ _ _ _ _ _ _ _ _ _ _ 79
Simplicity Is Key _ _ _ _ _ _ _ _ _ _ _ _ _ _ _ _ _ _ _ 89
Upgrades For a Healthier Life _ _ _ _ _ _ _ _ _ _ _ _ 95
Practical Tips for Wherever You Are _ _ _ _ _ _ _ _ 101
PART FIVE: PASSION _ _ _ _ _ _ _ _ _ _ _ _ _ _ _ 105
Lighting Up Your Fire _ _ _ _ _ _ _ _ _ _ _ _ _ _ _ _ 107
Awareness Without Attachment _ _ _ _ _ _ _ _ _ _ 113
Celebrate Everything _ _ _ _ _ _ _ _ _ _ _ _ _ _ _ _ 119
Conclusion _ 121
Acknowledgements _ _ _ _ _ _ _ _ _ _ _ _ _ _ _ _ _ 123
References _ 125
About The Author _ _ _ _ _ _ _ _ _ _ _ _ _ _ _ _ _ _ 127

INTRODUCTION

In 2011, I gave up the dieting game and finally lost the weight I had been carrying around once and for all. Losing the excess weight for good has been deeply empowering and totally freeing. No more conversations about being good all week, bad on the weekends, off the wagon, on a diet, feeling deprived, counting calories, making excuses or scrambling to lose weight for a special event. Letting go of all of this has brought such freedom and pure joy to my life!

I was never a chubby kid or overweight as an adolescent or young woman; however, as I got older, I never fully loved what I saw in the mirror, even before the weight started piling on. A bit of fat on my hips or on my stomach gave me reason to deprive myself of something I liked, usually chocolate or cake. This negative body image stuck with me and the dieting roller coaster kept me trapped for over 25 years, even for wanting to lose as little as 5 lbs.

In addition, stress played a big role in my life as early as when I was 20 years old. I was an over-achiever always striving for more. I had no idea that my body needed to be respected and appreciated, let alone how to do that on a regular basis. I thought it was a machine that would keep going forever. I would only stop when I was forced to because of exhaustion. This happened many, many times. My eating habits, stressful lifestyle and lack of respect for my own body led me to being 30 lbs. overweight. You know how we often need some kind of trigger for change, where we say enough is enough? Well, it took me three!

On June 8th, 2008 my mum died after being ill for 8 years. I made the trip back to England and, while at the funeral home in grief and trying to deal with the reality, I remember thinking about the saying *you can't take it with you when you die.* Suddenly this really meant something to me. It was very close and personal. Nothing that was important to my mum in the material world was going with her. It really affected me. I felt uncomfortable in some ways because it suddenly opened my eyes up to the reality of my own life. I asked myself why I was striving for so much at the expense of my own well-being. This was the start of making shifts in my own life.

Just 21 months later on March 14th, 2010 my dad died very suddenly. It knocked me sideways and it was more than I could bear at the time. I was only 46 years old and my parents were gone. The grief felt like navigating my way through thick fog and I felt even deeper confusion around the meaning of my own journey. The loss was huge and yet there were so many practical things that had to be taken care of. I made the trip once again from New York to England where I met up with my family. Not only were we dealing with grief and funeral arrangements, but this time we also had our family home and all its contents to deal with.

These two painful events stirred me up to changing my ways, but it truly took my own personal diagnosis to change the direction of my life. In 2011 it was discovered that I had two uterine fibroids. It took this diagnosis to admit to myself that permanent lifestyle changes were necessary and that I had to break away from just focusing on weight loss and to really focus on my health. I was given four options by my gynecologist. Three of them involved surgery and included a hysterectomy. The fourth was to do nothing. I was freaked out by this news. I had no desire to have surgery. I knew that I HAD to do something and I WANTED to do something to heal my body naturally.

I didn't realize at the time that these fibroids would be the catalyst for changing my life for the better and for good. They were a gift in disguise.

I started a hormone rejuvenation homeopathic program for three cycles that required a change in my diet and lifestyle along with using natural creams and drops. Giving up alcohol and eating as much organic food as possible was recommended during the program. I did both. I was afraid of what the alternative would be if I didn't deal with shrinking the fibroids or even worse, having them get bigger. The good news is that they shrank slightly and they continue to get smaller and smaller. The even better news is that I got healthy in the process and permanently lost the remainder of my excess weight.

My focus shifted from being obsessed about my weight and being consumed with a bit of fat here or a blemish there to truly becoming healthy. The transformation is amazing in so many ways. I no longer have weight issues. I have sustained energy throughout the day. I sleep well and I love taking care of myself.

The loss of my parents made me aware of my own mortality. I realized that we are here for a finite amount of time and I realized that my own health and happiness are the most important things to me.

My own personal diagnosis was the final trigger for creating permanent healthy changes in my life that I knew I needed, but until that point never really made happen. I stopped saying yes to everything and everyone, and I started to say yes to myself. I really started listening to what my body was telling me I needed. I still love to volunteer in various ways, but I don't take the lead and over commit to something if it takes away from taking care of myself. I do commit regularly to exercise, shopping for quality food and paying attention to the needs of my body.

I wasn't truly happy when I was striving for more and more and working every hour of the day. I was beyond stressed, overweight and not really living my life.

Now I am happy with the way I look and feel. I made changes that are lasting and feel like a joy, not a chore. I am thankful to my parents for the transformational gifts they unknowingly gave to me, and I honor them by treating my body with the respect it needs and deserves to thrive.

My journey has led me to helping other women ditch diets for good, find peace with food, focus on health and make themselves a priority.

I strongly believe the key to a healthy and happy life lies in the decision of every woman to simplify her life and focus on making herself a priority, instead of putting herself last.

Our health can't wait for us to be ready. And without our health, how can we enjoy and be productive in our lives?

Maybe you are frustrated with losing weight and gaining it back over and over. I was too. Diets aren't motivating and there comes a point when enough is enough!

Maybe you are fed up with having to buy larger size clothes. I certainly was. It's hard to feel sexy in something that you feel fat in.

Maybe you don't say or think wonderful things about yourself when you look in the mirror. I know I didn't. Even when I wasn't terribly overweight negative self-talk crept in. I remember turning over while having a massage and referring to myself as a beached whale and I would laugh, like it was out of my ability to do anything about it.

Maybe you play mind games with yourself by eating healthy during the day but binging at night while thinking that you are still eating healthy all the time. I did this all the time. It doesn't change if we don't become aware of it and face it.

Have you ever had your fortune told? Did you ever hear something that you didn't like so you went to a different fortune teller hoping for a different answer? Have you ever considered that diets are like this? We keep trying a different one in hopes of getting a different result but never realizing that maybe dieting is the real problem. Don't worry because I did too, but not anymore.

In this book I share with you what I call "The Powerful 5 P's for Permanent Weight Loss". It is my proven, solid solution for permanent weight loss and improved health. It is these 5 P's that led me to freedom from diets in 2011.

Before we get started, think about this - how can we make ourselves a *priority* if we don't change anything?

If we don't stop *pretending* about the truth of our lives, nothing changes.

If we don't shift our *perception* about how we see things, nothing changes.

If we don't have a *plan*, nothing changes.

And if we don't have *passion*, we are not interested nor committed and nothing changes.

So I invite you to keep an open mind and to welcome change, just like you welcome a dear friend you haven't seen in years.

"The Powerful 5 P's for Permanent Weight Loss" are how I naturally became healthy and how I ended the negative/frustrating food conversation that was taking up so much room inside my head and in my life. They have been a gift to me and I am gifting them to you. Please enjoy them and use them to your greatest good.

I am so excited that you are here and ready to take an inspiring and empowering journey to freedom from diets and to start living a life full of purpose and pleasure.

I have completely transformed my own life with this approach. My clients have completely transformed their lives and I know you can too.

My deepest wish for you is that you learn to value your body and health so much so, that nothing ever gets in the way of your most precious assets again – your health and happiness.

Join me as we Stop Dieting and Start Living, today.

Let's begin, shall we?

Part One

PRIORITIES

Life is a Balancing Act

What is this life, what is it for?
Should we do less, or should we do more?
What makes us lose, how do we win?
To have a good life, how do we begin?

All of these questions can run through ones mind.
Sometimes to the truth, we are so blind.
But it's time to shift, to change our perception,
And to get ourselves moving in a positive direction.

I'll tell you straight and I won't use tact,
Life is simply ~ a balancing act!
A life that's not balanced gets out of control,
It messes up ~ mind, body and soul.

Forget 'bigger is best' but don't think too small,
Don't tell a story too short or too tall,
Don't take too much, but don't live in lack,
Make it a balance, or you'll get out of whack!

Eat enough, but not in excess,
When you take that big portion, think about eating less!
Give to others, but I ask you please,
To leave room in your heart to also receive!

Allow others to help you, but don't be in need,
This is a message that I hope you will heed.
Embrace friends support and give it in return,
Being in balance is the best thing to learn.

The moral to this is to pick such a pace,
Throughout your life, which is neither to race
Nor to shuffle, but to be in perfect flow,
And living your dreams is all that you'll know.

Geri Jones — www.PomesByJones.com

Chapter One

ARE YOU MISSING FROM YOUR LIFE?

When I had to really get serious about my health back in 2011, the very first thing I had to do was start being kind to myself. All the changes I've made, all the benefits I have received, such as being healthy, losing the excess weight, and being free of pain or medications, came because of this simple, but very powerful thing, kindness to myself.

We often apologize to others for many different reasons, including not doing what we said we would do, forgetting a special event, or being unkind. How about doing this for yourself? Follow along with the letter below and see how you can start being kind to yourself.

Dear One and Only Body,

I am so sorry I have been ignoring you and your needs for longer than I care to remember. I really do love you even though I sometimes act as though I don't. I know I have been full of all kinds of excuses. It's so challenging with so much going on all the time. I honestly do want to put an end to my excuses and make time so you do your best as the precious gift you are. We both deserve that.

You see, the reality is I don't really see them as excuses because I have so much going on every day. In all honesty though, some of it is not a good use of my time! I get easily distracted and spend time on things that are neither productive nor enjoyable. If you were really in dire straits, diseased and needing treatments, of course I would make the time for you.

What have I been thinking? Why have I been making everything and everyone else a priority, instead of you? I am absolutely going to make the time

9

for you every day in a loving and caring way. No more lying or pretending that I am being good to you. It's simply just not fair to you.

I promise you that things are going to change starting today. This very minute. No more excuses.

I am not taking you for granted anymore. Instead, I choose to honor you and to show up for you every day, as you do for me.

I will charge you up every day just like I charge up my mobile phone. I'm sorry that I have considered my phone more important than you. I don't want to be without it and I don't want to be without you. I will "power you up" every day by giving you rest and plenty of sleep, so you are empowered.

I will fill you up with fuel that helps to get you around without any problems. I would never put diesel in my unleaded gas car because it would damage the engine, so why would I do this to you? I will give you the right kind of fuel every day and take care of you.

I will stop overfilling my days, weeks and months so that I have room for you. I would never try to overfill my blender or my suitcase when I travel so that it won't close, and you deserve the same. I declare today, no more overfilling!

I will make daily deposits of nourishing foods, love, and respect. I will think of you like my bank account. I make regular deposits so I can pay for my material needs, and I will do the same for you, so you have what you need to thrive every day.

I will simplify my life and get rid of the clutter to make you feel lighter and happier. I will clean up my messy home, my thoughts and my relationships. I will stop being lazy and take care of all my messes.

I am going to invest in you and get the help and support I need to make it a reality. I won't look for quick fixes anymore. No more diets, gimmicks, deprivation and the like. I will make taking care of you a lifestyle that we BOTH love and enjoy.

I am falling in love with you and my life just like when we were young, innocent children. We are going to have some fun!

Thank you for sticking with me through thick and thin.

I am so excited about enjoying healthier and happier days with you, and I know that when YOU and I are happier and healthier, EVERYONE gets to benefit from it!

Much love,

Yours Truly xoxoxo

Are You Missing From Your Life?

I know this might sound strange but have you ever considered that you might be missing from your life? You are nowhere to be found on a mental, physical, emotional or spiritual list of priorities. Have you ever had a conversation with yourself about this? Does it feel impossible, maybe even a myth to make yourself a priority? Yet if you don't, who will?

People do nice things for us at times and we feel appreciated from time-to-time, but what about the in-between times? When you make yourself a priority, the nice things from others become the icing on the cake. Bringing more awareness to your own needs and saying yes to yourself more and as often as possible doesn't mean suddenly becoming irresponsible and blowing off your commitments. It is simply about honoring yourself in a healthy way and acknowledging that you have needs and desires that deserve to be fulfilled, instead of leaving yourself on the side line. Think of it as showing up as the real, whole you, every day.

Our Patterns Form at an Early Age

I married two months before my 20th birthday, the first time around. In fact, at that time I was a wife, a step-mother of two, a godmother and an auntie. I was older than my years. I loved being married, having my own home and my own life. However, it was challenging with a ready-made family and so many responsibilities. I had a mortgage and money was tight. I often felt overwhelmed and stressed, but there were many wonderful times too. Even back then, it seemed normal to me to put everyone and everything else ahead of myself. I never even considered that I wasn't making myself a priority or deeply acknowledging my own needs and wants. During one of my periods of exhaustion from over-doing things and dealing with stress, my dad told me that only one person could change things. That person was me. He was absolutely right. I only made changes when I was forced to in order to feel better, but as soon as I was up and running again I was back to my old ways. A bit like having a hang-over and saying that we will never do that again – until the next time. We can quickly forget how awful we felt.

We form patterns early on in life that can end up staying with us for a long time, even our whole lives. We tell ourselves that all is well, but somewhere deep down and buried we know that something is missing. We even wear "masks" to show the outside world that all is rosy in our lives. Have you considered that you have patterns? What do the patterns of your life look like? Do they bring you happiness? Have you always thought you should take care of everything and everyone else no matter what? It's just "who you are," right?

Before we know it, the years pass by and we find ourselves in situations that we don't like in all kinds of ways. These patterns translate to how we show up in the world and how we take care of ourselves. Unhealthy patterns keep us from that true sense of feeling satisfied on a deep soulful level.

All too often, a diet becomes a pattern too. I don't know about you, but I have never been excited about going on a diet. If excess weight has been a struggle for you and dieting has been your pattern for losing weight, please don't beat yourself up. It's not your fault. The dieting industry is a multi-billion dollar industry and we are bombarded with the promise of the next one and the next one as the solution to our problem. All too often, the pattern of dieting can leave us feeling like a failure, miserable and stuck. However, there is an easier and more effective solution other than using diet after diet for weight loss.

Are You Listening to Your Body?

When we really pay attention to all the alerts from our body, we have an opportunity to course correct before things become dire, but all too often we are primarily focused on losing weight and not necessarily on our health.

The human body is so amazing. Among many automatic functions, it regulates temperature, the heart beats without us thinking about it, and it lets us know when all is not well. When something hurts, it's our body's way of communicating with us. It wants to bring our attention to something so we will make necessary changes. It's a truly amazing system. Yet it is often an inconvenience for us to feel pain and discomfort, so we ignore it or take a pill in order to keep going. All too often we don't take the time to stop and listen to what is really going on or why.

The pain or discomfort you feel is a cry for help from your body. If you are overweight and your knees hurt, your body is letting you know that it can't handle that much weight. Taking a pill for the pain is keeping you from listening to what your body really needs you to do, which is to lose some weight. I know it's a drag to think about losing weight, especially when you've done it over and over again by going on a diet. A pill seems like the easy solution, so you can manage the pain without changing anything, but is that what you really want? Do you really want to ignore the deeper desire you have of looking and feeling great long-term?

Yet, being kind to yourself means making it a priority to listen closely to the needs of your body, just like you would for a close friend or family member that needed your help. Think back to when a child or someone you love cried for help. Chances are you did all you could to help them. You didn't ignore them and hope they would stop asking. Your body is no different. It is letting you know that it needs your attention and help to make it happy and well so you feel great and content on a much deeper level.

If our car started making a weird noise when driving along, we wouldn't turn up the radio to avoid listening to it. Instead we take care of the problem to avoid ending up stranded on the side of the road. Yet, we go for years, sometimes decades, avoiding listening to the alerts from our bodies, our emotions and our needs and wants. We stay stuck in bodies and situations that we don't love.

Well, my friend, it's time to start listening. Really listening to your body and how it is crying out for your help. It can't wait any longer. It's time to prioritize your own needs, starting right now. That includes quitting using one more diet or quick fix for weight loss. When you feel healthy and strong, you are able to help other people in your life when they need help. But all too often, we put others' needs before our own and we lose the connection to ourselves and our lives. You've suffered long enough, it's time to draw a line in the sand and start listening to your own needs and make yourself a priority. You need to do this now because if not now, when? Before you know it, another year will be over.

Your Precious Body and You Are the Ultimate Best Friends

I spoke with a lady a few years ago who was frustrated with her weight. She had tried different diets, exercise plans, and various

approaches to losing weight on and off over the years, but she was still stuck and unhappy.

After we had been chatting for a while, I asked her when she last liked the way she looked and felt. There was a silence which I honored, but then I wasn't sure if I had lost the connection. So I asked if she was still there. She responded with yes. Then I realized she was crying and she was trying to compose herself so that I couldn't tell. This question triggered such sadness in her. She may not have even realized it in this way, but the tears revealed the hurt and disappointment that was buried deep down inside. She was experiencing a form of grief because she was sad by the loss of herself in her life. It was 23 years since she last liked how she looked and felt. She was working seven days a week and she knew that she wasn't making herself a priority. She was avoiding taking loving care of her body and soul by working so much in a job that kept her inactive for hours a day. This lady is not alone, as many women have ignored their own happiness and health for years.

It's hard to find the motivation to keep playing the dieting game again and again only to experience the same deflating results. It might seem easier to get distracted and ignore your own needs and wants, but they will keep popping up and hitting you between the eyes until you pay attention, so let's get to it and end the game today. Please don't let another day go by before taking back the reins of your life.

Just like my dad told me, there is only one person that can change your life. Until we give ourselves permission to change and reclaim ourselves we will always be looking for the quick fix, the next diet or some external fulfillment to take our minds off what we don't like about ourselves and our lives.

Take a moment to think about whom you love and respect more than you love and respect yourself. Perhaps you even take better care of your car than you do of your own self. Our entire being deserves and needs respect, love, care, attention, and healthy fuel to function properly in this world. If our bodies are neglected, ignored and running on empty all the time, there is absolutely no way that they can function properly, let alone thrive.

If we treated our friends in a disrespectful way, they probably wouldn't stick around and your body probably won't either. Remember, your precious body and you are the ultimate best friends. Take care of yourself in every way.

Scrambling at the Last Minute

Do you have a habit of generally putting things off until the last minute?

Have you ever got low on fuel and wondered where the nearest gas station is? Do you panic when the low fuel light comes on and wished you had fueled up sooner? I know I have in the past and then wondered if I will make it without breaking down.

Our bodies, just like our cars, are vehicles that we rely on and need to get us to where we want to go. Think about what happens if you don't take your car in for regular maintenance. Eventually the car starts to break down. It could start with an oil leak and then an electrical problem. Then suddenly one day, without warning, the whole engine seizes.

I frequently hear from women how they know what they "should" be doing, but they aren't doing it. As a result they feel tired, deflated and emotionally empty. They grab for something that gives them quick comfort and short-term pleasure, but it leaves them feeling guilty and like a failure. They tell themselves that it's too late in their life to have what they really want. They believe that it's all downhill after 40 for their bodies, their desires, their waistlines and their ability to feel good about themselves. Then they scramble at the last minute trying to lose weight for an event that is fast approaching because underneath the hopelessness, they really do want to improve how they look and feel. When we make ourselves a priority and respect ourselves there is no more last minute scramble. Every day is just another beautiful day in our life.

Juggling Too Many Balls

I ran myself ragged for years because I wasn't making myself a priority. I overextended myself so much that I often felt like I needed a life raft to save me at times, but I would just keep on going. I couldn't say no to things. Sometimes I didn't want to say no because I really wanted to say yes, even though I knew I didn't have the time without compromising something else, which was usually taking good care of myself. I remember in 2010 having my ironing board up for 10 days because I just didn't have the time to get to the ironing and I'm a person who gets things done. I knew things were pretty dire and that I couldn't keep it up. This was the year my dad died, I was President of my local Rotary club, and I was working in Real Estate, in addition to many other things I had going on. There were far too many balls in the air and I felt it affecting me physically, emotionally and mentally.

I have countless stories about how I kept so many balls juggling in the air at once. I bet you do too. I didn't know how to create a healthy lifestyle that would free me from the clutches of food and too much stress. I didn't know how to balance things in my life or even have the desire to make lasting changes. We think that if we just get through "this" then we will be "okay", but then life creates another situation for us to juggle again. It simply is not sustainable for our health or our happiness, so it makes perfect sense to declare ourselves a priority and put an end to the juggling act.

Remember the safety announcement on an airplane prior to takeoff regarding an emergency situation, where we are told to put our own oxygen mask on first, before helping someone else. There is a very good reason for this. If you try to put the oxygen mask on someone else first, you risk both of you not getting masks on in time. In order for us to be able to take care of someone else, we must first take care of ourselves. I hope this resonates deeply and is something that helps put taking care of yourself first into perspective so you cease being a juggler trying to keep all the balls in the air.

The Fairy Tale Syndrome

When we are young girls, we discover the charm and excitement of fairy tales. We soon learn as we get older that real life is not a fairy tale. Yet, we still hope for those fairy tale magical moments to happen in our own life. The years go by and we realize that no one is going to rescue us like in the fairy tales we are raised on. We realize that it's up to us to create the life we want and deserve.

Diets are a bit like fairy tales. They are the knight in shining armor that we hope will rescue us from our excess weight and struggles with food. Each time we try a different one, we hope it will bring us a happy ever after, but it never does.

Imagine your life feeling delicious, delightful and full of flavor without waiting for someone or something to rescue you. A life without pain caused from eating foods that create inflammation and discomfort in your body. No more pills for dealing with pain. No more yo-yo dieting or buying different size clothes after every feast or for a special occasion because nothing fits. Close your eyes for a moment and take a slow deep breath in through your nose and breathe out through your mouth. Imagine your life being just the way you've always wanted it to be and you are the one manifesting it. Stay with this feeling for a few minutes or longer and keep coming back to experience how good it feels.

How to Make Yourself a Priority

It all starts with making a simple decision to declare it so.

Everyone has an opinion about what you should do and how you should do it. But what do you think? What do you want and need to feel happy and content in your life? Do you want to stop juggling so many balls? Do you want to take off your "mask" and be the real you? Do you want to start paying attention to what your body and soul need to thrive?

Knowledge is a wonderful thing, but implementation is what leads to transformation. We all know that we should be eating our greens daily, reducing sugar and sodium, limiting or removing processed foods, eating as much fresh food as possible that comes from the earth and is preferably organic or at least free of harmful pesticides. But if we don't have an interest in doing any of it or a desire to experience the benefits and improve our quality of life, then nothing is going to change.

I invite you to think about making yourself a priority as a declaration of self-love and self-respect that will connect you to that deep desire that lies within you, which may have been ignored for longer than you can remember. We all do pleasant things for people we love and care about but what about ourselves?

Please, go to a mirror, look yourself directly in the eyes and declare that you are going to start doing pleasant things for yourself every day. It could be as simple as making sure you consume plenty of clean drinking water every day, or not skipping meals.

It might not seem like much or even feel strange at first, but making these simple shifts are the first step to making yourself a priority and really honoring your whole self. It will put the bounce back in your stride and give you a sense of empowerment because taking care of you is what ultimately matters. Then, making healthier food choices will start coming naturally to you, as an expression of your self-love and self-respect, as opposed to the old pattern of forcing deprivation, rules and restrictions of a diet on yourself.

It's time to start viewing healthier choices as an act of compassion for yourself. It's time to become best friends with yourself again, or even, maybe, for the first time.

Are You Missing From Your Life?

Action Step

Download and fill in the blanks of your new Stop Dieting, Start Living Manifesto "Dear One and Only Body" with your commitments – **www.DietFreeAndHealthy.com/bonus** Sign it and read it every day. This is a very powerful commitment to yourself. Place it where you will see it every day as a reminder of why you are focusing on yourself. You are a priority and you matter. Complete this before moving on to the next chapter.

Chapter Two

There Will Never Be the "Perfect" Time

Waiting for the "perfect" time to make healthy lifestyle changes a priority is like waiting to strike it rich by winning the lottery. It might happen, but it's a long shot. You have to be proactive on a regular basis to earn money and the same goes for your health.

For many years I felt like I was up against the clock rushing from one thing to the next. Appointments, errands, paperwork, work life, home life, volunteering, life in general! In fact, I used to rush around a supermarket with my shopping cart, list in hand and either walk at a very fast pace or sometimes break into a jog because it was something I often didn't have time for. I do get a giggle out of sharing that story because my life is so different today. Now when I go grocery shopping it feels special to me, sacred even, and not something I try to squeeze in as inconsequential. I also enjoy supporting local farmers who raise happy, respected animals that have space to enjoy their life. I shop at health food stores instead of supermarkets. This is a far cry from when I used to buy meat and fish in bulk from the wholesale store, not read labels, or even care because I wasn't invested in making time for taking care of myself on a regular basis. I considered grocery shopping a chore; one more thing on my long list of things to do.

I regularly buy my weekly groceries from a health food store, which is part of a 400 acre organic biodynamic farm about 40 minutes from where I live. It's a lovely scenic drive there and back with little to no traffic. It feels like I am going on a fun field trip! I often take time to soak up the energy there by sitting down and enjoying a piece of their freshly made organic pizza or a freshly made organic soup. I might also enjoy something from their bakery made fresh that morning, and all without chemicals and preservatives. The whole experience feels so yummy. They support local farms during the growing season and display the name of the farm that grew the produce. It's the only place I have seen this and I really appreciate knowing that my food travelled such a short distance to end up on my plate.

Would you love to experience a shopping trip like this where it's enjoyable and relaxing, where you feel healthier from just walking into the building, and where you aren't bombarded by aisles of choices that offer very little in terms of supporting your health? If you live in the United States check out www.LocalHarvest.org to see what is in your area. It's a really wonderful resource and one that I recommend often. A local friend of mine was so thrilled when she found a local CSA (Community Supported Agriculture) practically in her own backyard that was listed on this website.

Does Life Seem to Get in Your Way?

Do you ever catch yourself saying there are never enough hours in the day or that life just always seems to get in the way? That things are always standing between you and the things you want to do for yourself? Ever yearned for a more joyful experience grocery shopping and cooking, but feel they will always be chores to be completed as quickly as possible?

Do invitations to social events prevent you from ever finding the perfect time to start making healthy changes and make yourself a priority? Something just always seems to get in the way, or does it really? Is it just an excuse? There is a focus around food almost every month, so letting this get in the way, will prevent you from ever getting started taking better care of yourself. Super Bowl, Valentine's Day, St. Patrick's Day, Easter, July 4th, summer picnics, vacations and birthdays, Halloween, Thanksgiving, Christmas and New Year and more will happen year in and year out. I am all about having fun. We all enjoy a party or a fun celebration. I totally encourage you to have fun as often as possible, but stop waiting for the perfect time to start being kinder to yourself. Any time is a great time to get started. Act as if your life depends on it because the reality is, it actually does.

Finding Time for Exercise

I always enjoyed sports in school and even through my late 20's; however, through my 30's and part of my 40's, I was less interested because I didn't have the time for it. I only made time when I was in ramp up mode with wanting to lose weight or feeling guilty about not taking care of myself. Thankfully, this is no longer the case. I now view exercise as necessary for health and part of my self-care routine, and not something for maintaining my weight. This shift in focus has created a completely different experience which means I exercise regularly because it feels pleasurable and something I want to do and not something that I feel forced to do.

Life isn't going to get any slower or easier to manage without our intervention. In fact, the pace seems to get faster and faster. Our attention span is getting shorter. Information is coming at us faster than we can consume it. Extra time isn't going to magically appear to make the "perfect" time for implementing positive healthy changes. So, it's down to us to make the decision that exercise is a priority and necessary for feeling healthy and therefore create the time to do it. It doesn't need to be an hour at a gym. Make it work for you and not against you.

Taking the stairs instead of the escalator or elevator on a daily basis could be a starting point at your place of work. You could park your car further away from the store or building, or power-walk when doing errands. Simple things at home like using a jump rope, doing some sit-ups, running up and down your stairs, jumping jacks, or dancing your heart out are all great ways to start to get you moving. We often don't start something if it feels insignificant, but every little bit adds up to a lot in a short period of time.

Not only does regular activity strengthen your muscles and improve heart and lung function, but it can also reduce your risk of major diseases, stimulate the growth of new brain cells, and even add years to your life. Exercise is also a wonderful stress reliever. When I have been busy on a project, like writing this book, I have noticed how much more refreshed I feel by stepping back and taking a class at my local gym. When we exercise, our body releases the feel good chemicals called endorphins.

One of my lovely 60 year old clients had an exercise bike at home, but when we first started working together she wasn't using the bike because the seat was uncomfortable for her. She had already made some inquiries about a new saddle, but didn't have any success. She had pretty much ceased exercising until we discussed other things she could do. She liked to walk and so she decided to walk around the area where she lives. The couple of hills helped to elevate her heart rate and break into a sweat, but she missed her bike. So, she finally decided to buy a new one and sell the old one. There was no stopping her after that. She absolutely loves the new bike, which means she rides it regularly. All it takes is finding the right fit for us. When an activity feels uncomfortable in any way, we are not likely to do it and stick with it. We don't all like the same things, so explore what you enjoy and start there. I discovered that I like Pilates and it really has made a difference to my core strength. Making exercise a priority because you know it's good for you will become more rewarding when it is something that you really enjoy doing.

When you decide to welcome exercise into your life, like a long-lost friend you haven't seen in years, you will make the time because it's another way of saying yes to honoring yourself and that always feels great and empowering.

Take care of your-WHOLE-self by taking one step at a time. It's that simple. Say yes to exercise and to feeling well. Healthier choices can add years to your life and quality of life to your years.

Putting Things Into Perspective

If you were suddenly faced with needing surgery or treatment of some kind, you would deal with it swiftly because you would consider it a priority, right? There is simply never a perfect time to deal with these types of situations. They just have to be dealt with. Somehow the time that didn't seem available for living a healthier life by choice is suddenly available when an unexpected or unwanted event occurs. These unexpected and unwanted events provide reflection on what we are doing on a regular basis and really help to put things into perspective in our lives. They provide an opportunity to identify where we have been ignoring our own needs.

We would not ignore the need to pull into a gas station when we are low on fuel even if we are late for something. It is just not an option to skip it because we can't get to where we are going without the fuel to run the car. Yet, we don't hesitate to skip a meal or buy something totally devoid of any quality nutrition if we are short on time. Thinking ahead is better than finding ourselves in these types of situations. We avoid denying our bodies the quality fuel they absolutely need in order to run properly often under the misconception of them not being a priority.

I have found the best way for making healthy home cooked meals, time for rest and play, time for making sure that routine tasks such as paying bills, grocery shopping, or home maintenance, etc., is to schedule it like an appointment with my hairdresser, dentist or chiropractor. We don't just show up without an appointment with professionals. Approaching the things you want and need for yourself in this way makes it become a reality because you will not cancel on yourself at the last minute.

Go ahead and try it out for yourself, especially if the current use of your time leaves you short on time for things you need to do for yourself. If you are currently eating TV dinners, take-out, etc. on a regular or even semi-regular basis as a way to save time by not cooking a healthy meal at home, this is an opportunity to refocus and look at your life from a different perspective. These kinds of shortcuts are robbing you of your long-term health and happiness while keeping you stuck in the dieting game.

The Time Test

Let's take a look at where you are spending your time.

You might be surprised at what you discover, but remember this is a no judgment zone, so be totally honest. Progress is hindered when we let a bunch of negativity get in the way or have resistance to change. If you feel like you've never managed your time efficiently, then now is your chance. Think of me as your cheerleader, because I am rooting for you to embrace making positive changes and discovering that you CAN make it a reality.

The truth is we seem to make time for things that are interesting to us. I'm not suggesting that you give up everything you are doing, but rather to take a good honest look and see where you can start taking the first step. Even a baby step towards making a consistent commitment to how you prioritize and schedule your time will do wonders. As previously mentioned, you will need to put everything in your calendar so you are never out of time. The last thing you want to be doing is grabbing something to eat that is causing you to be dissatisfied with how you look and feel or, even worse, thinking about going on another diet.

What does a typical morning look like for you? Do you have a cup of coffee and watch the news for an hour? Read the paper? Get on the internet? Do you wake up late and rush out of the house without any thought around what you will have for lunch and dinner? Doing this results in not knowing what you are truly consuming.

What does a typical evening look like for you? Does cooking feel like a chore and not worth the bother for one or two people or too much work to feed more people? Do you sit down all night and watch TV or hang out on social media and munch away on your favorite snacks?

Or perhaps you are back in school or starting a new job. You are overwhelmed with all that you have going on in your life and wondering how it is all going to work out without you falling apart. Feelings of overwhelm seem to be prevalent in our society today, and it's a perfect reason to re-evaluate and re-prioritize how and where you spend your time.

Mapping out your week ahead and seeing an overview of what you have going on will really help you to stop waiting for the perfect time to make yourself a priority. When you make time for yourself and become a bigger part of your life, you naturally are a priority.

There Will Never Be the "Perfect" Time

Action Step

I put together a simple day planner worksheet you can use for scheduling your day. You can get it at:

www.DietFreeAndHealthy.com/bonus

Write down where you are spending your time and use the examples to help schedule your day to adjust to a healthier lifestyle. I recommend doing this before reading any further. Please do not skip this exercise. You will get an idea of where and how you can make changes. This is a really powerful life-changing exercise. Stop waiting for the "perfect" time and start creating time. Grab your day planner worksheet and make your schedule right now.

Chapter Three

RE-EVALUATING WHAT IS IMPORTANT IN LIFE

When Aide decided to work with me in early 2014, she was concerned about high blood pressure, high cholesterol, and she wanted to lose 15 lbs. She wasn't taking any prescription drugs and she wanted to keep it that way, but she knew she needed to address her diet to heal her body naturally. Food in general was something that didn't interest her. She didn't enjoy shopping for food, cooking it or really eating it. She ate just to satisfy hunger. If she could have eaten pizza for breakfast, lunch, and dinner she would because it was an easy solution for her. Even though she had a pretty good understanding of healthy eating, she never actually put the information into practice.

All that changed, and within one month she became a new woman. She completely changed her life because she was eager and hungry for a change that would nourish her mind, body and soul. After showing her how to cook a meal once, but make enough to eat two or three times and do it without getting bored, she started to look at recipe books, go online for recipes, watch cooking shows, plan her meals and keep an ongoing shopping list. She was ecstatic! Her blood pressure went from 131/86 to 110/73. She lost 10.5 lbs. She increased her exercise and she went from drinking a few sips of water a day to 7 glasses a day. The great thing is when she leaves her home, she thinks of her water container in the same way as her keys. She just doesn't leave without either one anymore. She is so thrilled with the results, and so am I because it has transformed her life. She continues to glow and she has now created a lifestyle that is simple, fun and enjoyable that supports her health and her weight. She basically stopped making excuses and jumped in with both feet because her health became of utmost importance to her.

Pulling Back The Curtain

I have met many wonderful women on my travels who have achieved success in several areas of their life including career and finances, but they still feel unhappy with how they look and feel and are hungry for a deeper sense of meaning to their life.

On a scale of 1 to 10 how happy and healthy do you feel right now? Have you been so busy over the years climbing the proverbial success ladder and building your material wealth, that you have ignored your own physical, mental and emotional health without even realizing it? If so, don't beat yourself up. Our society always seems to be pushing us to do more, have more and of course, use a diet for weight loss or a quick fix like a "magic" pill. If you feel like it's impossible to change the status quo and become a priority, don't despair because you are not alone. It's a common challenge; yet, it creates a sense of isolation, frustration and suffering in silence.

Sometimes the busyness of life can be a distraction and even an avoidance of looking at the truth of how we feel about ourselves and our lives, but deep down something keeps nagging away. Just take a moment now to pause and reflect on how you really feel and what has been important to you over the years that perhaps isn't as significant as it once was. Sit with it. Feel it. Breathe into it and make a deep connection to how you feel, perhaps for the first time or even in a long time, to how you really view your life in this moment and what is truly important to you.

If you feel sad and want to cry, just allow the tears to flow. A good cry is very healthy. I love a good one myself.

I spent years going after more and more at the expense of compromising my health and waistline, and it left me with the feeling of not being fulfilled on a deeper level. It wasn't just stuff. It was also personal achievements, awards, etc. I had a pattern of overextending myself. I never used to think of my body as something that was important to me in terms of my day-to-day life or something I would need in good shape as I got older. It was just my body. I didn't always like the way I looked, but thinking about whether it would break down or let me down wasn't something that crossed my mind until I was forced to stop due to exhaustion or illness. I took it for granted that my body would just always be there performing for me. I assumed that one day I would be able to kick back and enjoy the fruits of my labor. Your body is with you every second of every day whether you are in motion or asleep and it deserves the best of everything on a daily basis, not just when it's exhausted or screaming at you in pain to realize its importance.

Apart from the financial impact of becoming sick and the frustration of not being able to do what we want, it is such a worry for us and those that love us. Realizing that we are important and that we matter is another way to move the needle away from excuses and quick fixes and step into the life we want without excess weight, health issues, too much stress and aches and pains. We have to stop blaming everything and everyone else for our situation if we want a better life, including failed diets, and shift the focus on investing in ourselves. What we eat, drink and think all have an effect on our mind, body and soul. The question becomes, is having a wonderful healthy happy life important to you? I hope your answer is yes!

Your Goals And Desires

Most of us have goals and desires of some kind and that's a wonderful thing, but are they pie in the sky or realistic? Think about what your goals and desires are. They might be to run a marathon, raise money for a charity you feel passionate about, join a yoga class, a local gym, or grow your own food. Maybe you want to move to a new home, visit a particular place, or do a renovation.

Do you find yourself saying that you wish you could blank? If so, have you thought about why you haven't done it? Is it something that is realistic and attainable given your current circumstances or even a possibility in the future? If it is, that's great. Put it on the calendar. If not, put it on the back burner or strike it off your wish list, especially if it is causing you to complain, feel dissatisfied with your life and use food for comfort.

Does it really make sense to work an extra 20 hours or more a week to afford something, if it is costing you your health and happiness because you don't have time to take care of your basic needs?

Feelings of dissatisfaction often lead us to overeating or doing something that does not support our health and happiness and keep us in old self-defeating patterns. Letting go of things physically, mentally and emotionally creates an energetic shift in our own life as they free us from clutter. Doing this creates space and flow. When space is created, we are able to evaluate our life, our wants, our needs, our desires and find the answers to what is really important to us.

Re-evaluating What Is Important In Life

Action Step

The worksheet at **www.DietFreeAndHealthy.com/bonus** will help you choose one powerful action step to focus on what you can achieve for each time period in the next week, month, 3 months and 6 months. Put your focus on what you can make happen to make your weight and health goals become a top priority for you. Watch how things start to shift after doing this exercise.

Chapter Four

HAVING AWARENESS OF YOUR CHOICES

Have you ever been driving along and all of a sudden you reach your destination and you can't remember how you got there? I have done this many times and I think to myself, "Wow, I'm here already." We are like a plane on autopilot. Our mind is preoccupied with the list of things we have to get done or simply contemplating certain things, but we still make it to our destination even without being fully present.

Have you ever wondered if you washed your hair while taking a shower? Our minds wonder, but we still do things automatically that are routine to us.

Autopilot With Food And Drinks

Where in your life are you on automatic pilot with regards to your daily habits around food and drinks? Do you think you only drink two cups of coffee a day, have soda once a week or go out to dinner once a month? When I start working with a new client, I ask them how often they <u>think</u> they eat out. As things start to unfold, they realize that they eat out a lot more than what they thought because they do it automatically.

We can all probably attest to wishing we had made some different choices along the way in our life. If only we could turn back the hands of time and do it differently. Of course we can't do that, but we can learn from these types of experiences and make different choices going forward. Don't beat yourself up about things you have done in the past, whether it pertains to food binges, losing weight and gaining it back more times than you can remember, or anything else. The good news is we can choose a different path at any time and that includes letting go of dieting. You can start to build new habits around your food choices and make healthier choices a priority.

Know What You Are Eating and Drinking

Numerous times throughout my yo-yo dieting days, I drank a very well-known slimming drink as a meal replacement so that I could lose some weight. I never felt satisfied on it, but I just wanted to lose some weight. I had no idea back then about reading the ingredient list or the need to even check it. I used to think I was doing well. As long as I could lose weight, I was golden.

One of the big problems we face today is an industrialized food system. It looks like food, but is it really? So much of our "food" supply today is loaded with chemicals, pesticides and is genetically modified. We are also dealing with a new type of malnutrition. It's called processed food. It is no secret that the US is in the midst of a health crisis and things are getting worse, not better. But that doesn't mean we can't take responsibility for ourselves and learn all we can about what is going on, so we can take charge of our health, our waistline and our happiness. I believe in focusing on what we can change, and not what we can't change.

When I switched to removing much of the processed food from my diet and turned to eating organic foods, I felt lighter. My husband did too, so it wasn't just my imagination. We didn't feel bloated anymore. We were actually full and satisfied. It was a little strange at first because we were used to feeling full to the brim, or even over the brim sometimes.

It is so nice to eat quality food and not feel those awful uncomfortable feelings of bloating, gas and even nausea.

I strongly encourage you to know what you are ingesting and to become your own food advocate. Reading the nutritional label is not enough these days because of all the toxins contained in processed food. Learn what all the ingredients are on the label so that you know exactly what you are putting in your body and how it is affecting you physically beyond just changing the number on the scale.

Many digestive problems can be relieved just by having awareness of your choices and how you feel during and after eating. I have witnessed this for myself and with my clients when they become aware of what they are choosing to eat and drink instead of doing it on automatic pilot. I've seen how a healthier choice can relieve conditions such as Irritable Bowel Syndrome within a few weeks. It's so empowering and I highly recommend it.

Resistance to Change

Change is challenging for all of us. It does not necessarily need to be if we look at it through a wider lens.

If an 18 wheeler tractor trailer was heading for us, we would move out of the way as soon as possible to avoid the crisis of being hurt or killed. Yet, many food and drink choices are creating a different kind of crisis, albeit a slow motion crisis, as disease can and often does take time to manifest physically. Eating something loaded with chemicals isn't going to hurt us immediately, but there is a cumulative negative effect in the body.

One of my clients had purchased a whole batch of well-known weight loss products prior to working with me. When I looked at the packaging, I explained to her they were loaded with chemicals and harmful to her. She said she had spent a lot of money on them and she wanted to use them up, even though she wanted to lose weight and improve her health. If we were in harm's way in any other situation, we would move to safety. It's all a mindset shift. We have to be willing to make the different choices now so that we can reap the benefits going forward.

The more aware we are about the choices we make around what we consume, the easier it is to choose better quality products and the sooner we look and feel better.

Having Awareness Of Your Choices

Action Step

What's in your cupboards? What foods and beverages do you consume on autopilot that are harming you? Sugar and its various forms are the first place to start looking. As an example, High Fructose Corn Syrup is an inexpensive, overused, harmful ingredient found in so many processed products. The chart at **www.DietFreeAndHealthy.com/bonus** will help you bring more awareness to how your current choices may contain this and other harmful ingredients, so you can look for better options and still enjoy your favorite items.

Part Two

PRETENDING

Stop looking outside for scraps of pleasure or fulfillment, for validation, security, or love – you have a treasure within that is infinitely greater than anything the world can offer.

— ECKHART TOLLE

Chapter Five

WHAT'S REALLY WEIGHING YOU DOWN?

Excess weight isn't always necessarily just about poor diet and lack of exercise.

When I came to the United States back in May 1998, I wasn't planning to live here. I only came for three months on a visitor's visa. In July, just two months later, I met the man who would become my husband. We got married in December the same year and I started to make a life here. But I was so homesick. It lasted on and off for four years before it eventually lost its intensity. I had never been away from home for any extended period of time. I didn't realize it at the time, but this was really weighing on me emotionally. It ended up contributing to my annual weight gain because I was trying unconsciously to feel better by eating more, but it wasn't working and it was only adding on more pounds.

Exploring Possibilities

Our lives are like big jigsaw puzzles. Sometimes the pieces of our life seem to fit perfectly together and other times they don't. Let's take a look at the bigger picture of your life to see what could be weighing you down.

We have seen how, besides the lack of exercise and poor eating, there are certainly other areas in life that can contribute to weight gain, as in my case with homesickness, that you may not have considered. They are not necessarily all about emotional stuff, so let's take a look at some of these areas in your life and see where you can make some improvements that will help the excess weight come off without depriving yourself.

Clutter

Have you considered the clutter in your life and how you have been avoiding it, or even just ignoring it and pretending it doesn't exist?

Dealing with clutter is usually not high on the "To-Do" list for most of us because it doesn't feel all that appealing. If you have ignored it for some time, it can certainly seem overwhelming. Just knowing where to start can be a nightmare in itself. But, clutter of any kind can negatively affect your sense of well-being or shedding those unwanted extra pounds because it could be weighing you down.

Declutter Your Home

When you look around your home or office, how do you feel? Be totally honest with yourself.

Do you feel peaceful and calm, or do you feel irritated and uneasy? Do you see all the things that require your attention and then start eating for distraction and comfort? The pounds can creep on in the most unexpected circumstances and without even understanding why. Have you been meaning to file away papers, go through a stack of magazines or unopened mail? Have you been putting off organizing your closets because they are so full? How about donating clothes you haven't worn for over a year that perhaps still have the store tag on it. You bought it on sale just because it was a good deal, but apparently you didn't really need it because you haven't worn it. This has also happened to me in the past. What is lurking in your garage and preventing you from using it as intended? I bet you wish you could fit your car in there, especially on days when you have to scrape off the ice or remove the snow. How about the clutter in your car or your kitchen cupboards and refrigerator?

I'd wager that even having clutter behind closed doors is causing you undue stress and mental fatigue. And what about the things you have in storage units? This can also be a worry if it's a financial burden which can cause weight gain.

With so many demands on our time these days, you may be wondering how you can ever begin to address accumulated clutter. Such projects, whether big or small, take time and a plan of action to tackle them, but removing the clutter will have a positive effect on how you feel. Try it out for yourself.

Many people wait for spring-time to get to long awaited projects. We all know it as "spring-cleaning." After having the house closed up for months with windows closed and the heat turned up, it feels good to get the windows open and let some air in, doesn't it? We want to feel lighter and get going. Yet the truth is, we can clean up any part of our life at any time of the year we choose. I personally love to organize and spruce things up on a frequent basis. I really do enjoy it. It creates the physical sense of feeling "lighter" and being more in flow with my environment. The dead of winter on a snowy day is great for doing this.

I like to say, "Act like you are about to move at any moment." If you do eventually move, you will have less to do during an already stressful event. If you need help or accountability, ask a friend to help or hire a professional service. Stay in the flow, keep purging and decluttering and you will experience the benefits of feeling lighter in mind, body and spirit. You probably won't even give snacks a second thought as you get stuck in and start enjoying the process of cleaning up and clearing out and feeling lighter. Diets don't dig into these deeper parts of our life.

How To Start

If you feel like you don't know where to start, take a relatively small project like organizing a sock drawer and see how it makes you feel. You might find odd socks, worn out socks or just too many socks. Regardless, I know you will feel good about taking action.

Next, I encourage you to make a list of all the tasks that you want to accomplish. Start with the item that creates the most irritation for you. If it is a complete room, pick one area that you will start first. For example, if you want to start with your bedroom, you could choose the closet first and when that is complete, tackle the actual open space in the room. If the bedroom space itself bothers you more, start with that. Notice how your sleep improves due to the more tranquil energy you have created. Poor sleep can also lead to weight gain, so this is great motivation to start purging and cleaning up.

If your clutter has taken over, start with small steps. Taking a hike up a mountain begins with taking the first step. Focusing on the peak beforehand might stop you from wanting to walk to the top and miss out on enjoying the beautiful scenery once you get there. Pick one area of a room or one closet and start there. The changes aren't always so noticeable in the beginning, but as you keep at it, the rewards grow tenfold, and like the beautiful view at the top of the mountain, you will see how decluttering will bring more beauty, tranquility and flow into your own life on a daily basis.

Celebrate every accomplishment. Sit and have a cup of tea or something that you love that makes you pause and enjoy the moment and your work, like an artist stepping back to admire their creation. Praise yourself and really take a moment to let it sink in, to savor it, to appreciate it. This will add to the desire to go on with the next decluttering task and create a sense of joy rather than feeling like it's a chore.

Declutter Your Calendar

Unnecessary clutter that adversely affects our health also shows up in the form of over-committing ourselves in various ways, often leading to stress and weight gain. How does your calendar and schedule look and feel? Are you putting too many items on your list each day, only to either fail to complete them all or running yourself ragged trying to get them all done? Take a look at your commitments for the next week and see what you can cancel to give yourself more personal time. Ask yourself if you really want to do something or need to do it. We can easily get caught up by saying yes without thinking about how it will affect us. This was hard for me when I first made the decision to change my ways, but like anything else, it gets easier with practice.

De-clutter Your Mind

Our minds can so easily gather loads of clutter during the course of a day. This includes negative self-talk that prevents us from feeling joyful and alive, not feeling worthy or worrying about how we'll never get our life in order. Then there is the monumental list of things you have to get done. Making a conscious decision to slow down, smell the roses, and turn off the negative mental chatter is going to create space and have a positive effect on your life. When our minds are going 100 miles a minute, we are doing a disservice to our health and weight loss goals.

Excuses

We all have excuses in some shape or form, but are you letting your excuses run your life without even realizing it?

When I turned 35, I blamed my metabolism for my weight. When I turned 40, I blamed my hormones for my weight. At the time of writing this book, I am 50. I am not overweight anymore and I have never had a hot flash, but that could and probably would have been a completely different story if I had not made necessary changes to my diet and lifestyle. I never really thought about my life in terms of pretending or not being honest with myself, but when I finally stopped hiding behind my age as a way to shun self-responsibility and started being honest, things started moving in a positive direction. What is your excuse for what you don't like about yourself and your life? Are you blaming your age or something else? What are you pretending doesn't exist?

Getting Honest With Yourself

Are you a regular complainer, a procrastinator, a saboteur, a perfectionist, a martyr or something else in your life which has become a way of keeping you stuck and making excuses? It might seem "easy" to stay where you are or even impossible to change, but is it beneficial to you and really what you want at the end of the day? I'm guessing not. When we want something, we look for a way to make it happen. Sometimes the very thing that keeps us from what we want on a much deeper level can be a subconscious avoidance of the truth.

43

One of the most common excuses I hear about not making healthy meals is the need for recipes. So many women are convinced that they can't change anything until they find recipes. I call it an excuse because we can all find recipes on the internet these days. When they find one or two recipes they say they don't have time to make the meal, so the excuse transfers from one thing to another. This could be considered complaining or even procrastinating because there is no reason to be hung up on needing recipes and using that as an excuse to not eat at home more often. One of my clients had shelves stacked with recipe books, but she still believed that not having recipes was the reason why she was overweight. We often just want to put the blame on something or someone, but nothing changes if we don't stop pretending and really face the truth.

The second excuse I hear is one that has been placed on us by our society regarding menopause. We accept that we are doomed with never getting rid of excess weight or feeling great. It practically becomes a license to avoid making healthy choices and pretending that we have no control over our destiny. This belief serves no purpose. Start owning what you are doing and not doing. It will help to set you free from your struggles. A diet is not going to do that. Your excuses have a lot to do with your current reality if you are not looking and feeling your best. Take a moment to reflect on your current reality.

And the Truth Shall Set You Free

Cheating doesn't only come in the form of relationships. We also cheat on ourselves. I'm not talking about a structured cheat day where we go "wild" on Sunday because we have been "good" all week. I'm talking about the daily cheating that occurs that we don't want to admit to, which is a form of pretending things are different.

I used to play this game with wine. It became an all too often pleasure at the end of the day as a way to decompress. I would say I had a couple of glasses when it was usually 3 or 4. Other people didn't care what I did or didn't do, so why was I pretending to myself? Because I didn't want to face it, even though I knew it wasn't good for me in terms of my health and weight, and it negatively affected my sleep. I never thought of it as a problem because I wasn't thinking about it when I woke up or during the day. It was just my "treat" at the end of the day and I was worth it. I still enjoy wine, but I don't have so much or drink it so often. It's full of empty calories and was another big contributor to my weight gain.

What are you telling yourself? What story plays itself over and over? Do you tell yourself you are on a detox, but drink alcohol or eat out? Do you go to the gym, but don't break into a sweat because you aren't working hard, yet you think you're doing great because you are there? Do you eat food that you know is the direct cause of your pain and discomfort? Do you have a farm membership often known as a CSA (Community Supported Agriculture) or buy lots of organic produce at the store, but end up wasting so much of it because you eat out more than you eat at home? Do you procrastinate and say tomorrow or next week will be different? Do you get stuck in analysis paralysis? Do you blame the confusing and conflicting information about nutrition? Where are you not being honest with yourself?

When we play these mind games throughout the day, we are only cheating ourselves and preventing ourselves from having what it is we really want, which deep down is to be happy and content in all areas of our lives.

I know it often takes a lot to face the truth. None of us typically want to go poking around in our lives to uncover stuff we would rather pretend didn't exist. Yet, until we stop avoiding the truth about our reality, nothing will change and we will keep doing what we've always done and keep getting the same results we always have.

Whatever you admit to, be gentle with yourself. Please don't go on a guilt trip. It serves no purpose. Accept where you are. Be aware of where you are making excuses, and remember, no judgment or guilt allowed. As Suze Orman says regarding debt, "You have to face it to erase it." We can't change anything if we believe it doesn't exist. Are you ready to stop pretending and let the truth set you free from your excess weight once and for all?

What's Really Weighing You Down?

Action Step

Explore where you are pretending and not living in integrity. Do you usually eat a small meal and skip dessert when you are in company and binge when alone? Do you sometimes pay for things you can't afford to look good and suffer in silence over your debt load? Download this helpful worksheet:

www.DietFreeAndHealthy.com/bonus

The goal is to create awareness and become honest with yourself. You can do this. Go, Go, Go and commit, truly commit to completing this within the next 24 hours.

Chapter Six

WHAT ARE YOU REALLY HUNGRY FOR?

Until you discover the answer to this question, you will likely always struggle with food, excess weight and a life in some form of pain.

At the age of 30, I found myself alone for the first time. My marriage was over. It was my fault and I was a mess. I found myself filling my calendar so I didn't have to be alone with myself. Quite honestly, I didn't even know who I was. I had married very young and had huge responsibilities, which kept me from getting to know myself.

One night in my new single life, I actually said out loud to myself, "You are not going out tonight!" Something in me shifted. I knew I had been running away from feeling the pain about the reality of my life. I was scared. I didn't want to be alone. Everything that was familiar to me had come to an end. It certainly took courage to take a good honest look at my life and myself and make some changes. I can't say it was easy. It often never is, but it's necessary if we want to feel happy and content.

Keeping overly busy, looking for distractions consciously or subconsciously, and turning to something like food for comfort is so representative of being hungry for something much more than food.

We can run, but we can't hide. What are you running away from? Isn't it time to stop running away from what makes you unhappy? Discover what you are really hungry for and shed those unwanted pounds for good, without any deprivation.

What Is Food?

Food is really about nourishment and not just to satisfy hunger or be consumed as something to numb a feeling. Do you ever find yourself eating just for the sake of it and still not feel totally satisfied? I know I have many times over the years. You might feel so full physically from eating, but yet you feel empty at some level and you don't know why.

In my training at the Institute for Integrative Nutrition, I discovered that the food on our plate is known as Secondary Food and the food that fuels us on a more soul level is known as Primary Food. The Primary Food is often what is missing in our life, creating an imbalance. This is the reason why we turn to other sources of fuel in hopes of finding comfort and fulfillment. Unfortunately, all too often it keeps us stuck in patterns that don't serve us and we feel like a hamster on a wheel going around in circles.

Primary Food includes things like a happy home life, healthy finances, an enjoyable career, healthy fun relationships, doing exercise that you love, feeling expressive and creative, and experiencing joy in your life. The more Primary Food we receive, the less we depend upon Secondary Food and vice versa. The more we fill ourselves with Secondary Food, the less we are able to receive the Primary Food of life.

Feeling Full On Life and Not Just Food

Remember back to when you were a child playing, when you fell in love, or were working on a new project that excited you. Food was probably the last thing on your mind because you were satisfied at that much deeper soul level. Food never seemed to rule my world when I was younger. Yet as we get older, it can become like a virus growing in our minds that quickly takes on a life of its own. Interesting, isn't it?

As we go through life, it can become easy and even habitual to bury our head in the sand and pretend that we are happier than we really are. We may not embrace the truth of our despair about aspects of our life, including food. There are times in our life where we hide from ourselves, from others and from our truth. We don't want to show the "real us" in fear of not being accepted and liked by others or even worse, by ourselves. We think we are alone, but in reality there are so many people suffering with the very same thing. The longing to feel fulfilled on a deeper level and break free from the drama of diets is something I have seen over and over again in my coaching practice and from listening to conversations in general.

One of my clients felt like she wasn't very creative. Like me, she loves book work and administrative-type activities rather than drawing or painting-type activities. I will never forget, after a few weeks of making delicious, simple home cooked meals, she was so excited to realize that it was a way of being expressive and creative. She had never thought of it like that because when we first started working together, she was convinced she didn't like to cook and therefore, never had this experience. Now it's something that brings her joy and feeds her soul regularly because making food has become her Primary Food.

We need to start being honest and stop pretending and find the root cause if we want to lose the weight for good and find freedom from yo-yo dieting. Taking a look at the Primary Food in all areas of our lives is such an eye-opener and a fabulous starting point to discovering a whole new life free of diets, rules, restrictions and the misery of excess weight. It is often where we find the gold, the deeper meaning of our life and the truth about what we are really hungry for.

To start getting to know yourself on a deeper level, ask yourself what you are really hungry for. What triggers you to eat when you are not physically hungry? Triggers come in many forms, such as boredom, feeling down, anxiety, stress, worry, or loneliness. Does your job, your relationships, your home life, your social life, or anything else trigger you to eat when you are not hungry?

Taking a look at this is not a one-time deal, but rather regular assessing and tweaking. You may find that your patterns have been repeating themselves for decades. That's okay. Don't stay looking in the rear view mirror. That would be considered dangerous when driving and it could be of detriment to your deepest desires for yourself in your life. Keep looking forward. What if you shared your story of struggle with someone rather than just resorting to the same old approach of denial or a diet? I know you are not alone even though you may feel alone. How many more years will you hide from yourself? It just takes one person to start the conversation. Will you be the one? A lack of Primary Food is keeping you hungry. Bring awareness to this and watch the pounds melt away as you start to let go of what isn't working and embrace more of what you really want.

What Are You Really Hungry For?

Action Step

There is a term called "Bolting" that I discovered from Geneen Roth during my holistic health coaching training. When we don't want to feel something, we bolt and grab something that will make us feel better. Any time you feel the need to grab your favorite "go-to" as a means to change how you feel, stop, take a few deep breaths and ask yourself what you are really hungry for. It is very powerful. You might not change right away, but you will have more awareness for when it happens again, and as we know, awareness is the key to any change.

I have created a simple form with examples for you available at: **www.DietFreeAndHealthy.com/bonus**

Chapter Seven

Why Diets Don't Work

*The definition of insanity is doing the same thing over and
over again, but expecting different results.*

— Albert Einstein

Resorting to a diet for dealing with excess weight time and time
again is representative of being stuck in a pattern without any promise of
discovering freedom from the drama. This is because diets don't usually
address anything other than weight. They don't deal with our relationship
with food. They don't cover our relationship with our own life. There are
some diets based on a certain philosophy such as the Macrobiotic diet.
However, in general diets do not address anything to do with what is
lacking in our lives on a deeper level. This often leads us to use food to
self-medicate. Overeating is the symptom and not the cause.

Diets, by definition, are something that we go off. There is a
beginning and an end. The characteristics of a diet make them inherently
unable to work: it's not something you embrace for life; therefore, it can't
give you a lasting result. We don't think about it like this when we diet,
but it's one of those simple truths that holds so much power in creating a
shift in perspective.

Losing weight often seems like a challenge and a chore because the
approach seems too mechanical and restrictive and there is no fun in that.
The yo-yo pattern is often the result of feeling too restricted and once

51

you've reached your weight goal, as you have probably experienced, you'll be returning to your old habits and pack the pounds back on.

Why Does Your Own Metabolism Thwart You?

Simple, says Kelly Brownell, M.D., director of the Rudd Center for Food Policy and Obesity at Yale University: "The body may perceive dieting as a threat to its survival. It might not know the difference between Atkins and famine."

"What's more," says Brownell, who coined the term "yo-yo dieting" in the 1980s, "weight cycling can actually change your physiology. So the more diets you've been on, the harder it becomes to lose the weight. A hunger hormone called ghrelin increases, and a fullness hormone called leptin decreases, so you feel hungrier and less satiated."

According to research done by O, *The Oprah Magazine*, 80 percent of people who lose weight gain it right back. When I met Ann in January 2013, she was eagerly trying to lose 10 lbs. prior to going on a beach vacation later in the month. Like so many of us, she had tried numerous different diets over the years without long-term success or finding freedom from excess weight, so once again she was in that awful place of trying to lose the extra pounds to feel confident in a bathing suit. Since she felt time was of the essence, she had already adopted the 17 Day Diet in hopes of losing the weight quickly. However, like so many of us, she was incredibly tired of being on another diet. She knew as well as I did that she wasn't going to end the struggle of shedding the excess weight through using the "diet du jour" to solve her problem.

Every diet is a diet just with different wrapping. I gave her some pointers about what she could do to switch her thinking about focusing on losing the weight since she didn't want to start working with me prior to going on vacation. She knew she wanted to learn how to make healthy choices a lifestyle, so she could end the madness of dieting. Ann became a client upon her return from vacation and finally ended her relationship with diets. She now has so much more awareness about what her body really wants and needs instead of what her mind tells her she wants. Food is nourishment and enjoyment, not comfort or punishment. Ann is officially divorced from diets and I want the same for you.

We Are All Unique

During my holistic health coaching training, I studied over 100 dietary theories. Many diets are born out of something working successfully for the founder. They are anything from a few minutes, days and hours diets, calorie counting diets, anti-aging diets, parts of the body diets, percentage diets, names of people diets and ancient principles diets. The list goes on and on.

What works for one person won't necessarily work for another even if it is considered highly nutritious. Our digestive tracts are unique. Our body composition is unique; therefore, so is our body's response to what we eat. You may have an intolerance to a certain food, but a close relative is perfectly fine with that same food. So how can a diet "a one-size fits all approach" be the answer? It isn't. Even if you are not on a diet, serving the same meal to an entire family can cause digestive issues for some and not others. I have experienced this in my own home. Simply put, it is a question of finding what works for us individually so we focus on creating a healthy lifestyle rather than being concerned with counting calories, points, or anything else. If something upsets your system and feels uncomfortable, don't pretend it doesn't exist in fear of having to give it up. There is often a healthier alternative.

Diets often create a disconnection from listening to the needs of our body because the main focus is on losing weight and not on being healthy. When the emphasis is just on weight loss, we miss out on so much in terms of health and awareness of what our body is really asking for.

When I finally started living a healthy lifestyle and kicked diets to the curb for good in 2011, I realized that my obsession with weight gain often kept on the extra weight.

What we give our attention to is what we manifest. Once I let go of being obsessed about losing weight and I focused on being healthy, it no longer took up so much of my energy and it melted away.

Why Diets Don't Work

Action Step

Make a promise to yourself that you will never go on another diet again. Become aware of how much room food takes up in your head and let it go. Like any new habit, it takes time for it to become natural. Stick with it. Keep telling yourself you are so worthy of having a healthy body and a life you love. You don't need a diet for that. Keep looking at your new Stop Dieting, Start Living Manifesto every day to remind yourself that you are committed to being a priority in your life. If you haven't downloaded and printed out your copy of the manifesto then go now and do that before reading any further. It is the foundation for creating a body and a life you love free of deprivation, rules and restrictions.

www.DietFreeAndHealthy.com/bonus

Part Three

PERCEPTION

The Flying Trapeze

— An excerpt from *Warriors of the Heart* by Danaan Perry

"Sometimes, I feel that my life is a series of trapeze swings. I'm either hanging on to a trapeze bar swinging along or, for a few moments, I'm hurdling across space between the trapeze bars.

Mostly, I spend my time hanging on for dear life to the trapeze bar of the moment. It carries me along a certain steady rate of swing and I have the feeling that I'm in control. I know most of the right questions, and even some of the right answers. But once in a while, as I'm merrily, or not so merrily, swinging along, I look ahead of me into the distance, and what do I see?

I see another trapeze bar looking at me. It's empty. And I know, in that place in me that knows, that this new bar has my name on it. It is *my next step, my growth, my aliveness coming to get me.* In my heart of hearts I know that for me to grow, I must release my grip on the present well-known bar to move to the new one.

55

Each time it happens, I hope—no, I pray—that I won't have to grab the new one. But in my knowing place, I know that I must totally release my grasp on my old bar, and for some moments in time I must hurtle across space before I can grab the new bar. *Each time I do this I am filled with terror.* It doesn't matter that in all my previous hurdles I have always made it.

Each time I am afraid I will miss, that I will be crushed on unseen rocks in the bottomless basin between the bars.

But I do it anyway. I must.

Perhaps this is the essence of what the mystics call faith. No guarantees, no net, no insurance, but we do it anyway because hanging on to that old bar is no longer an option. And so, for what seems to be an eternity but actually lasts a microsecond. I soar across the dark void called "the past is over, the future is not yet here." It's called a transition. I have come to believe that it is the only place that real change occurs.

I have a sneaking suspicion that the transition zone is the only real thing, and the bars are the illusions we dream up to not notice the void. Yes, with all the fear that can accompany transitions, they are still the most vibrant, growth-filled, passionate moments in our lives.

And so transformation of fear may have nothing to do with making fear go away, but rather with giving ourselves permission to "hang out" in the transition zone -- between the trapeze bars -- allowing ourselves to dwell in the only place where change really happens.

It can be terrifying. It can also be enlightening.

Hurdling through the void, we just may learn to fly".

Chapter Eight

CHANGE YOUR PERCEPTION
AND CHANGE YOUR LIFE

An old friend of mine told me many years ago that during her lunch break with her co-workers the majority of their conversation is about losing weight and not being happy with their bodies. They think because they have reached "that age" in life this is how it is going to be for the rest of their lives, always trying to find the next best diet or talk about what they will cut down on or give up completely! Don't you just love how society conditions us to expect certain things to happen at certain times in our life? So many women are consumed with the topic of food and excess weight and at some subconscious level they feel safe being with each other and sharing the same problem. They have created their own private mini "let's stay stuck in the problem" group without even realizing it.

Then of course there are larger organized group meetings where you get weighed and measured and praised if you have made improvements. I'm familiar with these because I have attended them. I never really liked them personally, but I know others who do. It felt like a crutch, but I didn't know why at the time. Looking back it can become a place of camaraderie and socializing; therefore, subconsciously it's something we don't want to end. At some level it keeps the problem in play. After the meeting, many go out for dinner and eat foods that are totally unhealthy and lead to weight gain! It just doesn't make any sense, but they are all in the same boat and it feels safe.

We can't expect our bodies to be there for us if we don't take care of them. Women often come up to me like I am the "Food Police" and start telling me how well they are eating, but the reality is something is "off" because they don't look the picture of health.

Are you willing to make some changes by changing your perception so you can set yourself free?

Managing Symptoms

When you change your perception about what it truly means to be healthy instead of just slimmer, you will naturally want to make healthy changes in your life. I regularly hear from women about their thyroid issues and how they have been told by their endocrinologist that they have to be on the medication for life and they take that advice without any consideration of shifting their perception towards thinking of an alternative approach. One lady told me she has been on medication for her thyroid problem for 15 years and it has caused damage to her liver. The liver is the janitor for the body. The body cannot maintain health with this constant pollution of chemicals from medication, yet taking pills to manage symptoms has become the norm. The problem still exists if the symptom is being managed. This is what diets do. They manage a symptom, instead of addressing the cause of the problem. This is why they can't set us free.

I personally dislike taking pills. For one, I can't swallow them, so I have to crush them up and two, I am afraid of what they are doing to my body. There are certainly times when medicine is a lifesaver. If I found myself in that situation I would think differently, but taking it daily or for extended periods of time doesn't feel natural to me. I don't even have a painkiller in my home. A hot water bottle and pure essential oils are two of my regular natural first-aid friends along with alternative therapies such as acupuncture, massage, reflexology, chiropractic and energy work.

When I was in my mid 20's, my car was smashed up by two men with baseball bats while I was sitting in it with my ex-husband and his young son. We couldn't pass their car on a narrow road and the next thing they were outside of their car and attacking ours. Needless to say, it was horrific. I ended up with post-traumatic stress and a prescription for valium from my doctor. I took one pill and didn't take any more. I don't know why I didn't use them as a crutch, but somehow I knew that I had to deal with the trauma in order to heal it and not mask it. I was frightened to drive to work in the daylight. I experienced being paranoid for many months because my sense of safety had been violated. It took a year to truly heal from the trauma, but I did it without pills.

Are you willing to inquire about getting off your medications? The body can be very forgiving if given half a chance. Shifting your perception about making necessary dietary and lifestyle changes from the viewpoint of long-term health rather than short-term weight loss or disguising symptoms is a simple approach to improving the quality of your life.

It's a pity that the natural holistic approach to health has been termed as "alternative" and yet many years ago people turned to nature for cures to ailments. If you want to get off your harmful medications start looking at the "alternative". As Hippocrates said, "Let food be thy medicine and medicine be thy food." It may take some time to safely transition away from medication, but being a team player with your doctor and being proactive is a smart move. Let your doctor know you aren't interested in a prescription for the rest of your life. I am very proactive with my medical doctor during my annual physical and I recommend you are too at each and every visit.

Portions Out of Control

I never had huge meals growing up. It just always seemed to be the "right" size and there were never any leftovers. My mother cooked just enough to feed all five of us, but we often had some kind of dessert both at lunch and dinner. In the early days of my life in the States, I would often ask my husband if he wanted the American or English version of a sandwich. He actually was happy to have the thinner English version. It always seemed to me that the meals in the US were enough to feed three or four people! Before I knew it, I was used to eating more and it became the norm for many years.

During working with one of my clients, she was frustrated that the excess weight wasn't coming off quickly enough. She did have a thyroid problem, but with changes in her diet her thyroid was back in normal range within 3 months. That was fantastic news! She made many positive changes including eating dinner earlier, not snacking late at night, buying organic food, eating out less, and cutting down on sugar, dairy and gluten. So, the detective in me knew that something was still off. Finally, she said that she needed to cut down on her portion sizes. Bingo! That was the missing piece and the weak link in the chain. You see, her perception was that she had made so many wonderful changes, which she had, but she had missed embracing a vital piece of the puzzle, portion size.

Bigger portions mean we eat more than we need, so consider using a smaller plate or bowl as a way to transition from overeating from larger portions. This will help to shift your perception from thinking you are being deprived if you only have food on half your plate instead of it being completely full. In my home, we typically don't use plates for dinner anymore. To help us feel fuller longer, we use a bowl instead and take more time to eat the meal.

We are overconsuming in many areas of our lives today. We often don't need as much of anything as we think we do, whether it's food, clothes, furniture, gadgets, etc. When we have more room on our plates, in our closets, or in our homes, we tend to fill them up just because there is room. It's certainly something to ponder over. Where in your life are you overconsuming?

Fear of Change

Changing your life for the better is about being willing to do the right thing for you even when everyone else is doing it differently.

Do you talk and act like you want to lose weight permanently without being on a diet ever again, but deep down inside you are afraid of what it will mean if your friends or partner don't do the same if they have the same struggle? Where will you belong? Will you be lonely for a while? These are certainly genuine concerns and valid thoughts, but the truth is that *not having what you most desire* is having a negative impact on you at a much deeper emotional level and can keep you feeling in a rut. Remember what we discussed in Chapter 6. The more we deprive ourselves of our Primary Food, the more we fill ourselves up with Secondary Food.

Who Are You Spending Most of Your Time With?

Let's say you were successful and you finally got to your desired weight and looked fabulous. There could be jealousy on the part of the others you hang out with. There could be fear on your part that you will no longer "fit in" because you aren't "like" them anymore. Have you considered that this fear could be a reality that is keeping you stuck?

What do you think would happen if you decided once and for all that you were going to break the cycle of dieting and really start focusing on what the underlying problem is, so you can switch your perception about your excess weight and get rid of it once and for all?

I encourage you to be yourself, your true self. Step up and make a stand for what you really want and who you really are. If you don't want a piece of cake because it's someone's birthday or you're with friends and family for the holidays, then don't have it. If you don't want to have another drink because someone says one more won't hurt you, don't have it in order to keep the peace and fit in. How many times have you allowed people to force their views and opinions on you only to end up feeling frustrated and annoyed?

I remember experiencing this very situation when I was on the hormone rejuvenation program for the uterine fibroids. I was so committed to shrinking them and doing everything I could to improve my situation that I stayed firm. At that point I wasn't concerned about being on a diet in the way I had for many previous years, I was focused on my health and I lost weight as a natural side effect. A simple shift in perception to not worrying about what others think is what contributed to changing my life for the better. You can change yours, too.

The True Cost of Convenience

When I was living a fast-paced, stressful life, I became less and less interested in cooking at home. It seemed like a chore and I frequently wasn't interested in whipping up a meal. It was not uncommon for us to eat out four times per week on average. My husband didn't really feel like going out after working all day in our landscaping business, but if I didn't have a meal ready we had to go out or pick something up. It just seemed so convenient not having to deal with preparing a meal and the clean-up at home.

I didn't have the awareness then that I do now, but the fact is when we eat out we are not really sure what it is that we are eating. It often tastes good and we all rave about a great meal and a great experience at a particular establishment, but we don't often know the quality of the food, the distance the food traveled to end up on our plate, whether it has been genetically modified, or whether the animal had a happy life or miserable life, in a factory farm pumped with hormones and antibiotics. All these things are important because they contribute to our overall health and how we look and feel. I didn't really know that I wasn't feeling great until I made changes in my life and started to feel better. Health isn't the absence of disease, it's a state of complete physical, mental and social well-being. Health is living free of ongoing issues and without medication to manage symptoms such as headaches, constipation, anxiety, stress or fatigue. These symptoms are not labelled as diseases, but they are signs that health is compromised and often get overlooked until they become more serious and lead to disease.

Processed foods seem very convenient, don't they? They save us time and that is something you may be short on these days. We have three types of foods in our society today: plant based food, animal products, and processed foods. Processed foods are being consumed in huge quantities and are a major contributor to the declining health of millions of people and the rise in obesity. They are often loaded with harmful chemicals, a lengthy ingredient list and words that are hard to pronounce. You may have heard the health conscious mantra popularized by Michael Pollan: "If you can't pronounce it, you shouldn't be eating it." Have you ever read the label on your bread? How many ingredients are in it and how many can you pronounce? Ever wondered why it can last for weeks without going moldy? Food is not supposed to be immortal. That's why we had many bakeries years ago.

Do Your Own Due Diligence

A processed item that is often touted as healthy is almond milk. Carrageenan can be found in processed almond milk found in a carton. It is a common food additive that is extracted from red seaweed, *Chondrus crispus*, popularly known as Irish moss. Carrageenan, has been used as a thickener and emulsifier to improve the texture of many products such as ice cream, cottage cheese, yoghurt, soy milk and other processed foods.

Although carrageenan is derived from red seaweed, a natural source, veteran carrageenan researcher Joanne Tobacman, MD, associate professor of clinical medicine at the University of Illinois School of Medicine at Chicago says, "Carrageenan predictably causes inflammation, which can lead to ulcerations and bleeding." Her previous work showed a concerning connection between carrageenan and gastrointestinal cancer in lab animals, and she's involved with ongoing research funded through the National Institute of Health that is investigating carrageenan's effect on ulcerative colitis and other diseases like diabetes.

When we switch our perception about the way we view convenience, we realize there is a huge hidden cost associated with it because the build-up of toxins and chemicals will likely lead to the inconvenience of becoming sick or even worse, contracting a life threatening disease. It doesn't take long to make a nutritious home cooked meal. All too often it just comes down to thinking ahead and perceiving it as an act of kindness to ourselves.

Nutritious or Non-Nutritious

Many times when I initially meet with a client for a VIP session, they will ask me to write down a list of foods that are good and bad. I tell them that I don't view food that way and I recommend that they don't either. We all seem to learn in childhood how things we do are considered either good or bad and these descriptive words stay with us for years and are often used as labels to describe food. We also learn that if we are "good" we get a reward. If we are "bad" we are punished.

When it comes to food, one of the liberating things you can do for yourself is change your perception of food being good or bad to being nutritious or non-nutritious. It removes the judgment around it. We associate with negative thoughts when we think something is bad. It can send us down a negative spiral very quickly and the behavior continues to perpetuate keeping us stuck. For example, fresh steamed vegetables are more nutritious than vegetables from a can. A sweet baked potato is more nutritious than French fries. You get the idea?

Change Your Perception and Change Your Life

Action Step

Commit to being true to who you are and what you want. When you are in situations where people are forcing their views and opinions on you, just stand your ground. If it feels uncomfortable at first, don't worry. Keep on doing it until it eventually feels natural to honor yourself and what you want. Putting it on your radar and having the awareness is the first step to creating a healthier life for yourself. One way to stand your ground and honor your needs is to make healthy alternatives that you can share with others.

I have made a video to show you just how quick and easy it is to make your own healthy almond milk that is free from carrageenan, so you never have to buy the harmful, ready-made version again. You can download the recipe at:

www.DietFreeAndHealthy.com/bonus

Chapter Nine

GIFTS COME IN MANY FORMS

(GIFT – *Get Inspired For Transformation*)

We associate gifts with something fun and joyful, such as birthdays and the holidays, but have you considered that gifts may come in the form of a negative or painful experience that initially has you running for the hills?

I shared with you that the arrival of uterine fibroids flipped me out when I initially got the news from my gynecologist, but I soon realized they were a gift. It wasn't a typical gift beautifully wrapped and given to me for a special occasion. It was an unexpected gift in disguise. Without them I may still be a yo-yo dieter, facing a challenging time in menopause and not feeling well in general. I realized that I was changing the course of my long-term health and the quality of my life. I didn't want to follow in my mother's shoes just because we are told that certain things are hereditary. My mother started menopause at age 41 and she had a terrible time. She even ended up with cancer in the lining of her womb. This led to a hysterectomy and a subsequent nervous breakdown. Her health continued to decline at some level from there. Don't get me wrong, there are still days when I feel challenged with things going on in my life, I am human after-all, but they are fewer and farther between. When things crop up, I look at the deeper meaning and revisit the Primary Food in my life and reach out to the closest people in my life who understand me for support and reflection. It's not always easy to see things as GIFTs in the midst of a challenge, but a little space and time can change our perception.

Where are your unwrapped GIFTs hiding? What events have happened in your life where you still feel resentment, anger, or let down? What if you revisited these events and looked at how they might have been a gift in disguise? How would your life be different if you actually embraced the experience as part of your journey and an opportunity for personal growth? Eating junk and dealing with weight issues could be the direct result of not accepting an experience or event as a GIFT leading you to **G**et **I**nspired **F**or **T**ransformation.

Shower Yourself with Gifts

I enjoy giving and receiving gifts and you probably do, too. I love that feeling when I get just the right gift for a person and it makes them happy. It feels so good. How about showering yourself with gifts that make you happy on a daily basis? There are so many gifts you could be giving to yourself on a regular basis that don't cost you a penny or need wrapping.

Giving yourself little gifts throughout the day and making sure that you are being kind to yourself feels so delightful. I like going to the movie theater by myself sometimes very spontaneously on a rainy afternoon. It feels like a simple gift that makes me happy. These simple gifts can be drinking a glass of water as soon as you wake up. Not skipping meals. Declining an invitation and not committing to something if it will put you under pressure. Taking some food with you when you know you will be out for a few hours or more, so you eat something healthy, instead of stopping for nutrient deficient food that will negatively affect your health and weight. Unplug from technology. Take in the scenery. Enjoy a sunrise or a sunset. Smell the flowers. Remember in the old days that Sunday was a day of rest? It seems like a lifetime ago.

Life is beyond fast these days. Declaring that you are going to start giving yourself these simple yet powerful and effective gifts is a beautiful, empowering, delicious act of self-love.

The Gift of Laughter

My sister was diagnosed with HER2 breast cancer in February 2013. I was so upset when she told me, and I was afraid for her. We cried on the phone together. We were like this as children. When one of us was hurt, the other one would cry.

I went to visit her in France in August 2013 after she was finished with chemo, but still going through radiation. It was hard to see her in such rough shape with no hair and her right breast removed. It brings tears to my eyes as I write this. I did many things to help out including making wholesome meals, gardening and rubbing her feet. However, the one thing that seemed to be so uplifting for her was laughter. She told me that I am really funny. We ended up actually having quite a few belly laughs.

One morning while I was weeding the vegetable garden, I heard a noise coming from the house. I wasn't sure what it was at first, but as I got closer I realized it was the vacuum cleaner. She hadn't been able to personally use it in months, but she told me she was feeling so much better because of all the laughter. What if you saw having fun and a good old belly laugh as a gift to yourself and others because it improves how you feel? It is so healthy and healing and it doesn't cost a penny. It helps to shake things up and shake things off. Just like a dog having a whole-body shake. This is one of the gifts we can give to ourselves and others daily. Even several times a day if we so choose. It is so therapeutic.

I highly recommend changing your perception about how to improve your current situation by simply showering yourself with daily gifts. They will all contribute to feeling great and finding freedom from excess weight. What could be better than giving yourself the ultimate gift of health?

Gifts Come In Many Forms

Action Step

When we improve our own life, we automatically improve the lives of others. It has a domino effect. Please visit **www.DietFreeAnd Healthy.com/bonus** to download your free guide to help identify where you can begin giving yourself GIFTs in your life that bring you meaning and a smile to your face.

Chapter Ten

INTEGRATION, NOT SEPARATION

I've lost track of how many times I thought my New Year's resolutions would be the cure-all for losing weight. It gave me a license to go wild and eat and drink what I wanted over the holidays, because when the New Year rolled around everything was going to be different. New Year's Day was the silver lining after all the madness of over-indulging, over-extending and over-spending was over. Sound familiar?

Separation Mentality

How many times have you finished up all your junk foods and said, "This is it, this time will be different," and then stopped off somewhere to buy what you were craving and ate it in the car because you felt deprived? I have more than once. Just because it didn't make it into your home, you tell yourself that it didn't happen or it didn't count. So removing everything that is unhealthy from your home isn't the solution for getting healthier and slimmer. Isn't that refreshing news!

When we feel deprived, our mind won't shut up until we give it what it wants. I see people beating themselves up all the time because they made a "bad" choice and they feel they "fell off the wagon" again. I was caught up in this for years too, but it really saddens me to see so many people struggle because it doesn't have to be this way. The problem is it's a separation mentality which leads to feeling like there is no escape. I used to think I had two choices: either eat what I wanted and deal with the weight, or be on a diet and feel deprived. I too had separation mentality instead of thinking about integrating the junk until I could phase more of it out of my life gently and without force.

The more you become invested in transforming your life instead of worrying about excess weight, the more you will naturally make healthier choices and switch from focusing on it purely from a weight perspective. The goal is to see every day as just another day, a lifestyle where your choices are an integrated part of your life. Therefore, it doesn't matter what time of the year it is. You relax and enjoy life because you are no longer thinking in terms of this or that. You are embracing it all instead of fighting it.

This is one of the reasons I don't recommend a detox to someone who is not invested in making healthy choices on a regular basis as a way of life. It can do more harm than good in some cases and it often leads to craving the foods that were missing during the detox, leading to binging. It totally defeats the purpose of cleaning out the toxins in the body.

I tried detoxing for the first time back in the year 2000. I couldn't last a day! But now, because I love giving myself daily gifts of healthful foods etc., it is a pleasure to do a detox because a lot of what I consume on the detox is what I am consuming in my regular diet which is juices and blends. This gives the digestive tract time to relax from breaking down food after we swallow, as it is predigested and it feels like real food, because it is. I don't feel deprived. I don't have side effects such as headaches and feeling worse before I feel better because I don't have an overload of toxins in the first place. I also don't believe in detoxing for extended periods of time like 21 days or more and I stay away from buying a "system" of products and pills. Keeping it as natural as possible is my approach. When we view our choices around food from an integrated standpoint in our daily lives, it is no longer something that feels difficult or separate from us. A detox can be viewed as another gift because it clears out any cobwebs and brings about a sense of peace, calm and clarity.

The holiday season, vacations and special events are huge triggers when we don't have an integrated approach to our daily lives around food.

If excess weight and dieting have been part of your life over and over, I encourage you to think about this integrated approach. It really is life-changing. Whether I am at a party, a graduation, a networking event or anything else, I hear at least one woman say how she is depriving herself of something and happy to be losing weight on a diet that works "this time". I know it's all a game because I have played it many times. I am so glad to be done with these games and you can be done with them, too.

Integration and Implementation

How many times have you gone to a workshop or seminar and felt inspired to implement what you learned, regardless of whether it was how to better manage your money, manage your time, a spiritual workshop or how to eat better? We've all left these events feeling pumped and ready for change. All too often though, just like New Year's resolutions, it becomes something that we don't do for long. We don't know how to integrate it daily, so we lose interest and momentum. This can lead to feeling deflated because it didn't turn out the way we wanted it to. We may even blame the teacher or presenter for not providing enough information to actually make it happen for us, but the buck stops with us.

When it comes to embracing new ways of eating and living, don't try to figure out everything in the first week or you will likely discontinue. However, if you think of it in terms of a life-long commitment with simple baby steps taken regularly on an everyday basis, you will be invested in gathering not only the information, but also remain committed to integrating and implementing and overcoming any obstacles or challenges.

Our bodies change over time and what seems to work today may not work in the future. Being mindful of listening to the needs of your body, detaching from all the hype about the latest dieting trends and false marketing will keep you grounded and connected to living every day in receiving mode and making the best choices to support your overall health and happiness.

<u>Integration, Not Separation</u>

<u>Action Step</u>

I've provided a list of baby steps you can take to implement on a weekly basis. Choose three to get started and implement others as is appropriate for you and in a timeframe that feels right. You can download the list at: **www.DietFreeAndHealthy.com/bonus**

Chapter Eleven

INVESTMENT OR EXPENSE?

The cost of health care in the US is astronomical. Some people have literally gone bankrupt as a result of needing surgery or any type of ongoing medical care. The sad part is that so many of these health problems are a direct result of poor food choices in terms of quality and quantity, and could have easily been avoided. It is less expensive to eat well than it is to get sick. Prevention is cheaper than cure and a shift in perception about what really constitutes an expense can really turn your health around.

How many times have you purchased something that you couldn't afford, but you bought it anyway because it was what you wanted? Perhaps it was a large purchase like a car, a vacation, or a new appliance, clothes or eating out on a regular basis. No matter what it was, if you decided you wanted it, you found a way to purchase it.

What are your thoughts when it comes to buying quality food? It's true that organic food costs more at the register than conventionally grown, genetically modified, pesticide laden foods. But, is it really an expense or is it an investment towards being healthy?

Have you considered how much you spend on daily purchases of coffee, snacks, lunch, dinner, take out or alcohol? Keeping track of these types of expenses for one week will be a real eye-opener.

Someone told me once that they were spending about $1800 a month on eating out because they were so busy and didn't have time to cook. Imagine how many fabulous healthy organic groceries that would buy. Yet, all too often the perception is that quality food costs too much money. Switching your perception about price will go a long way towards feeling better. Take a look at where you are <u>actually</u> spending your money and where you <u>could</u> be spending it if you want to look and feel better.

We typically buy what we want and not always what we need. Yet what our bodies really need is a break from the over-processed, artificial chemicalized junk that acts like an intruder in the body, robbing it of vital resources.

Your Body is Like Your Bank Account

If you made regular withdrawals and no deposits from your bank account, sooner or later, likely sooner, you are going to wind up in the red. Well, your body is just like that and when you keep requiring it to provide you with energy withdrawals, but you aren't putting in healthy nutritious deposits, you are going to bankrupt your body.

We all know that eating vegetables in their original fresh form are great for enjoying good health, yet they are the number one food missing from the modern diet. Learning to incorporate quality vegetables, including dark leafy greens, into your diet is essential to establishing good health and keeping your body out of overdraft and becoming sick and diseased.

Changing your perception about the price of quality food that feeds your body and soul might take some time, but including organic greens in your diet is a great place to start. Nutritionally, greens are very high in calcium, magnesium, iron, potassium, phosphorous, zinc and vitamins A, C, E and K. They are loaded with fiber, folic acid, chlorophyll and many other micronutrients and phytochemicals and are a high-alkalizing food. Knowing this is all well and good, but I would love for you to actually experience it in your body. It will elevate your mood too because food does affect your mood. Try it for yourself.

Put yourself BACK IN CHARGE of your life and health and start thinking of your health like your bank account. Is it healthy or deficient? Is it worth switching your perception to thinking about your choices as investments? I believe so!

<u>Investment or Expense?</u>

<u>Action Step</u>

I've created an eye-opening interactive spreadsheet to help you determine where and how you are currently spending your money on food and beverages. It shows how you can take that information and apply it to budgeting for healthier foods. To download the worksheet please visit:

www.DietFreeAndHealthy.com/bonus

Part Four

PLAN

If you don't design your own life plan, chances are you'll fall into someone else's plan. And guess what they have planned for you? Not much.

—JIM ROHN

Chapter Twelve

PROGRESSION, NOT PERFECTION!

Both my parents were perfectionists about everything they did. They saw it as taking pride in everything which they considered a positive thing, and they raised their children to do the same. Perfection could have been my middle name! I used to worry about getting every detail perfect or waiting for the perfect circumstances. This would sometimes stop me from taking action. My first desire for writing a book was 20 years ago when I found my spiritual path and started to discover who I am. I wanted to help others who felt lost to find their path, but I thought who would want to listen to what I have to say. How would I get started and what would I include in the book? After all, did I really have enough to share with the world? I thought other people who were leaders in this field, who were my mentors, were better than me. I regularly compared myself to other people, which stopped me from making a plan to go after things I wanted. I didn't believe I could have it or do it. Can you relate in some way? All too often my perfectionistic mind created self-imposed obstacles that would hold me back instead of just taking the plunge. This left me feeling angry and frustrated.

This pattern of perfectionism and not feeling good enough has played out numerous times in my life. Now I am aware of it; I don't allow myself to get stuck in it. It really isn't my friend like I thought it was growing up. So, here I am taking imperfect action and writing my book from my heart, stepping out and sharing experiences even if it isn't perfectly written because I care about helping you transform your life and shed the excess weight for good and getting healthy in the process, like I did. If I waited for it to be perfectly perfect, it would never get into your hands and you would miss out on a completely different approach to looking and feeling better. A friend of mine used to say, "Perfection is in imperfection!" I totally understand that now, but it took me years to get it.

Some of my clients have said to me they will never be like me. I say, "That's good, because I am me and you are you!" They see how I walk my talk and have reached a point where living a healthy lifestyle comes naturally and easily to me. As you know, it wasn't always that way. In this situation, I am the mentor and they are the student. They get concerned with doing everything "perfectly" to impress me. I can totally relate to that, but it's not about perfection. It's about progression. This is how we get the ball rolling. We just say yes to ourselves and get started from where we are.

I stayed on this path because I didn't concern myself with doing everything perfectly. I was definitely committed and I still am, but that doesn't mean I live my life in a straight-jacket. I focused on my health because I wanted to rid my body of uterine fibroids and this naturally translated into losing my excess weight for good without a diet. I viewed the changes I was making as a life-long journey and not a short-term goal of weight loss. This is this reason I talk about focusing on progression and not perfection. We all need to go wild from time to time and trying to be perfect all the time can lead to feeling like a failure if we don't conform to the standards we have set for ourselves. We all need to live our lives at the end of the day the best we can. I am certainly well-travelled along the "diet free and healthy path" at this point and it feels fabulous to be free of having to lose weight over and over again, not feeling deprived, free of any aches and pains, and not taking any prescribed medications. You can have all this too, but you have to get started and let go of trying to be perfect.

Taking the First Step

When a baby takes its first step, it is a wonderful sight to see. They are so excited and pleased with themselves and in a very short period of time they are taking more steps. Then they get into everything as their world becomes more interesting and they start exploring as much as they can. Taking on something new in our lives such as a new lifestyle and eating healthy food is the same thing. We are simply exploring new territory.

Taking the first step and then the next is called progression, just like a baby learning to walk by taking one step at a time. A baby isn't concerned with perfection or thinking about a finish line when they start to walk. They just naturally start the process of learning to walk. Quitting the dieting game and making healthier choices all start with taking the first step which naturally evolves into a new lifestyle. If you fall, just like a baby does at first, get back up and take the next step from where you are. A baby doesn't give up and you don't have to either while learning something new. Be curious about where these steps will take you. They will open up a whole new world of possibilities, a sense of freedom and a deeper meaning to your life where you feel confident making plans for things you haven't done in years.

The All or Nothing Syndrome

During a VIP day with a new client, whether in person, on Skype or phone, I never suggest they remove <u>everything</u> from their cupboards that is having a negative effect on their health and waistline because it's too much too soon. I don't want them running for the hills and giving up before they get started. The mere mention of quinoa (keen-wah) to someone who has been living on potato chips, cookies, and fast food could send them in a spin. I still identify the harmful culprits, so they are aware of them. For someone who is eating less processed foods, we dive in a little deeper. Either way, we always create a plan of action. A plan becomes a reality.

Let's take a look at where you can make some adjustments that will have a huge positive impact in your life. I encourage you to keep reminding yourself to take one step at a time, and just keep moving forward. This makes it feel doable and a lot more fun. Before you know it, you will be making better choices because it feels natural and not forced. It will be on your terms and not someone else's.

The Seduction of Sugar

Sugar is not only something that affects your waistline, but it also has a detrimental effect on your health. Excessive sugar intake can lead to type 2 diabetes and create inflammation known as the "silent killer". It may increase the risk of osteoporosis, certain cancers, high blood pressure and other health problems. Sugar is added to many commonly consumed items, including all kinds of soft drinks and it is hidden in almost all processed foods.

Many sugars end in "ose" and include: Sucrose, Maltose, Dextrose, Fructose, Glucose, Galactose, Lactose, High Fructose Corn Syrup and Glucose Solids.

However, there are a lot of sugars that don't end in "ose" that you should be aware of. Such as: Cane juice, Barley malt, Caramel, Date sugar and Malt syrup. For a list of harmful sugars, please see the action step worksheet in chapter four.

The single largest source of calories for Americans comes from sugar — specifically high fructose corn syrup. Just take a look at the sugar consumption trends of the past 300 years taken from www.Mercola.com:

- In 1700, the average person consumed about 4 pounds of sugar per year.

- In 1800, the average person consumed about 18 pounds of sugar per year.

- In 1900, individual consumption had risen to 90 pounds of sugar per year.

- In 2009, more than 50 percent of all Americans consume one-half pound of sugar PER DAY—translating to a whopping 180 pounds of sugar per year!

It just keeps getting higher.

Planning to remove sugar completely from your life is going for perfection. Don't set yourself up for failure. I don't know anyone who has quit sugar permanently and you don't have to. It is certainly considered progression and a step in the right direction to start paying attention to how much you are consuming, so start there. Keep in mind that 4 grams equals 1 teaspoon of sugar. Take a look at one of your products now and figure out the sugar content. It is shocking!

The video Death by Sugar **www.DietFreeAndHealthy.com/death-by-sugar** is a great resource that shows how much sugar is hidden in the foods we commonly eat. It also provides an example of how sugar immediately negatively alters our blood and overall health.

Another way to understand how much sugar we put in our bodies is to really see how much is in a single item. When I am speaking to a group or coaching privately, I put the actual sugar total amount contained in soda into an empty soda bottle for demonstration purposes because it is such a strong visual. We have to literally see it to wake us up. It is not uncommon for a small soda bottle to contain 12 teaspoons of sugar. Is it any wonder we have a health and obesity crisis?

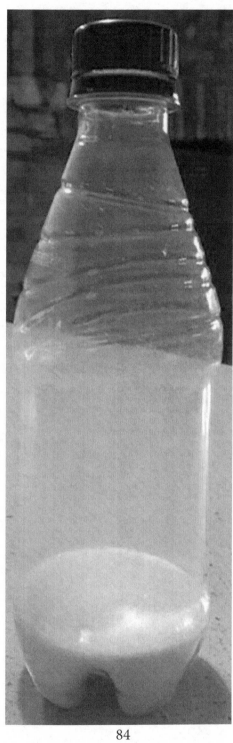

The Wonders of Water

Most of us are aware of the importance of drinking plenty of water. Getting our daily requirement of water helps us in so many ways, including organ function, keeping skin clear and hydrated and allowing physical action in the body to flow smoothly. Yet, many people find it just as challenging to drink enough water daily as reducing their sugar intake. Having a plan of action is the first step in the right direction!

The general rule of thumb is to half your weight and then divide by 8 to determine how many 8 ounce glasses of water to drink per day. If you are 200 lbs., this example would equal 12.5 glasses of water. I know that might sound like a lot. If you are not used to drinking water this may seem impossible to do, but it could also be too much too soon for your kidneys to handle. Start out slowly by perhaps having up to half of this amount and monitor how many times you are going to the bathroom. If you are constantly urinating, you may need to back off until you have adjusted. You be the judge and plan accordingly.

I personally like the taste of plain water, but you may prefer to add lemon, lime, mint or something similar. However, this is not an excuse to put artificial flavor crystals or sweetener in your water. Consuming enough water is often easier during the warmer months. During the cold months, I put my daily requirement into a pitcher instead of trying to keep track of the number of glasses I drink. This way I know I am consciously trying to get my quota for the day. Some days I don't drink as much as others, especially if I don't get started early enough, but I still drink plenty. If it doesn't come naturally to you, then it will require some planning. Drinking too much prior to bedtime could interrupt your sleep, so paying attention to this will help you figure out when the best time is for you to stop. For me, it's at least two hours before going to bed.

Avoiding Dehydration

The signs of dehydration in adults range from minor to severe and can include: dry mouth, poor digestion, sluggish thinking, skin breakouts, bad breath, thirst, dry skin, headache, constipation, low blood pressure, or generally feeling tired and more. Many of these ailments disappear when more water is consumed. A friend of mine once told me she suffered from regular headaches. I told her it was probably dehydration and to drink more water. She said she drank lots of water. I know that "lots of water" is very subjective. When I asked her how much, she said 3 glasses. That really isn't enough. When she increased her water intake, the headaches went away.

When I tell people that I don't have any pain medication in my home, they ask me what I do when I have a headache. On the rare occasion that I do get one, I tell them that I go through a mental check list. Have I drank enough water that day, am I tired, am I stressed, or do I need a chiropractic adjustment? Remember, pain is the body communicating with us informing us that all is not well. So many symptoms disappear as a result of drinking plenty of water on a daily basis. When a baby cries, it is informing the parents that it needs something such as food or a diaper change. Once they have been satisfied, they stop crying. Drinking plenty of water is a way to satisfy the cries for attention from your body.

When I initially spoke with Rona, a client of mine, about drinking more water, one of the simple shifts she made was to put her water on a small table so it was at eye level rather than on the floor next to where she was sitting and out of sight. This was a perfect solution to drinking more water. If it is out of sight, it is out of mind.

Drinking an adequate amount of quality water is a must for staying hydrated, so plan what will work for you. Think about where you are throughout the day and where you can have water placed. It definitely takes some conscious effort at first. I take water with me in the car. I have a glass at my desk. I have a glass by my bedside and I have a glass where I sit in the living room. To get you started, schedule a reminder in your calendar. So for example, at 10 a.m. "drink 3 glasses of water by noon" but also remember to have a glass of water as soon as you wake up. Decide right now what your plan is for making sure you drink plenty of water.

Know the Quality of Your Drinking Water

I used to have a reverse-osmosis system on my water at home until I discovered that it removes all the minerals from the water. Because it lacks minerals, when it is consumed, it also leaches minerals from the body, which means that the minerals being consumed in food and vitamins are being urinated away. This, of course, is not good for our health. One popular trend involved adding minerals back into the reverse osmosis water, but according to the World Health Organization, possibly none of the commonly used ways of re-mineralization could be considered optimum, since the water does not contain all of its beneficial components. Be sure to know the quality of the water you are drinking at all times and do any necessary research. Read the ingredient list on bottled water. It isn't always just water! Some restaurants and other public places have chlorine in their water. If I smell it, I don't drink it. Become committed to drinking the best water you can.

Progression, Not Perfection!

Action Step

I use a very simple system for tracking daily sugar intake. I put it together for you in a spreadsheet available at:

www.DietFreeAndHealthy.com/bonus

Chapter Thirteen

SIMPLICITY IS KEY

If you can't explain it to a six year old,
you don't understand it yourself.
— Albert Einstein

I grew up in a very simple home environment. We weren't over-indulged, but all our basic needs were met and then there were a few treats as well. My parents generally kept things simple. My mother made simple meals and often had the same menu week after week. My sister and I would run to catch the bus home from school and knew what was for dinner by the day of the week. We weren't always thrilled, and although my mother would switch it up a bit from time to time, it wasn't very often. She liked routine a lot, as she found it made life easier, and we always ate by 5.30 at the latest. They had simple routines, simple values and simple pleasures. My dad used to actually say that he liked to keep things simple. If things did feel like they were getting out of control, he would make everything simple again as soon as possible.

When he died very suddenly, it was no surprise that everything from a legal standpoint was in order. If you have been in this situation, you know that dealing with the personal belongings of deceased loved ones is very hard. It was so comforting to us that their simple approach to life resulted in very little being thrown away.

My parents kept their home neat and orderly. They had a place for everything, and everything in its place. They were very practical and they didn't overconsume.

Over recent years, I can really see the value in living a simple life, but for many years I wanted more because simple seemed too uninteresting for me. I wanted more excitement and more things. There is nothing necessarily wrong with wanting more, but not if it comes at the price of feeling overextended, miserable and unhealthy trying to afford it to keep up with the Joneses. The short-lived euphoric feeling we experience from buying something new, leads to an emotional crash. It leaves us feeling like we need something else so that we can experience that feeling again, and so the cycle continues. We end up becoming over consumers and life suddenly becomes complicated by wanting more and more.

The Ease of Simplifying

Many people are craving a more simple life today, but don't necessarily know how to make it happen or where to start. So, they end up staying in overwhelm and overload.

Simplicity is a journey and not a destination. I have done a lot to simplify my life, such as not overcommitting myself and making myself a priority, but I feel a desire to do more. I used to love the pressure of a deadline or be up for a challenge when I was younger, but I don't like that feeling anymore. The older I get, the less I want to deal with things that clutter up my mind, emotions and life. Are you feeling the same way?

Simplifying Your Kitchen

One of my clients has childhood memories that the kitchen was such a mess with stuff all over the counter tops, dishes in the sink and spoiled food in the refrigerator which prevented her parents from making healthy family meals.

It became a challenge in her own adult life to find the motivation to make healthy meals until she said enough is enough and got organized.

Having a kitchen that functions well is a beautiful thing. Keep it cleaned up and uncluttered after every meal. It's hard to start preparing and cooking a meal when you have to clean up from the previous day before you can get started.

Do meal planning on the same day each week for the week ahead so you have the food in your kitchen when you need it.

Take inventory of what you have and what you need.

When will you make it?

How will you get organized?

How often will you go to the store – every day, once a week?

Addressing these details will simplify your life an incredible amount, making it easier to cook healthy nutritious meals made with love. For motivation on including more real food in your diet, take a look at the trailer for the video documentary called *Forks Over Knives*, **www.DietFreeAndHealthy.com/forks-over-knives**

One of my favorite recipe books is called *Raw Food Made Easy for 1 to 2 People* by Jennifer Cornbleet. It is such a simple book as many of the recipes use a lot of the same ingredients. The meals are simple to make and require very little time and clean up. I hardly ever follow a recipe, but this book has become one of my all-time favorites. Find one or two recipe books that you like and get rid of the rest if you haven't used them in ages and they are collecting dust. A simple uncluttered kitchen functions best.

Simplifying Other Areas of Your Life

When you bring your mail into the house, go through it the same day. It sounds so simple and yet many find themselves overwhelmed because it piles up so quickly. Just taking a few minutes each day will keep things manageable and uncluttered.

Create a simple filing system, if you don't already have one, to avoid getting frustrated and annoyed when you are looking for a document. It doesn't have to be anything fancy. I used to have a concertina file in my early 20's, so I could always find what I was looking for. Something as simple as putting all your household appliance manuals in one place will simplify your life when you have a question about an appliance. Writing the date of purchase on the manual will take the guess work out of trying to remember how old it is. It's so simple and effective, but it might not have crossed your mind.

Unsubscribe from email lists that do not interest you or serve you anymore. I do this regularly. We all get bogged down by too many emails these days and it can lead to feeling like you are drowning in a sea of overwhelm. I would love to stay on some of the lists, but the truth is I just can't read everything that comes my way, so unsubscribing and dealing with less emails makes life more simple and happy.

Check emails and the internet two or three times a day at specific times. I know this is a challenge for most of us, including me. But, I do turn down the volume on my computer so I can't hear the arrival of a new message when I am focusing on something. We are more productive when we are focused and less stressed.

Make a list of everything you do. I did this once and I filled up 4 pages of a small yellow lined pad. I included everything from watering indoor and outdoor plants and laundry, to making appointments with contractors, running errands and dealing with the mail. I couldn't believe how much I wrote down. It was no wonder I felt like I was doing too much. All the small day-to-day things add up to a lot and create overwhelm. Seeing the full picture will help you see where you can simplify or even plan to delegate some of the tasks.

Trying to live in the here and now is a wonderful way to simplify, but it is so much easier said than done. When we worry about anytime in the future, whether it's an hour from now or next week, it can bog us down and create a sense of overwhelm which negatively impacts how we feel.

Step away from overconsuming the news. I know a lady who stress eats over what she hears on the news. If this triggers you to eat more, make a simple decision to limit viewing time or unplug altogether. We all have a choice.

Plan to travel lighter next time you go somewhere. Many of us take too much stuff when we go places. When I visited my sister in France in August 2013, I stopped to see my family in England first. My suitcase was so heavy that I could barely get it up and down stairs or on the escalator. The airline even placed a sticker on it cautioning to bend your knees before picking it up. It was such a nuisance and I declared that I would never do that again.

Make time for self-reflection and self-nourishment. It doesn't have to be a huge chunk of time each day, but the key is to actually do it. Keep it simple and doable and plan for it.

Being healthy makes life simpler. Being unhealthy is complicated and can take so much time with managing doctor's appointments, prescription refills, tracking the times to take the pills, etc.

When we stop and look at all areas of our life, we really do find many ways we can start simplifying. It makes us feel lighter in mind, body and soul.

Simplicity Is Key

Action Step

Use the commitment form at **www.DietFreeAndHealthy.com/bonus** to identify the areas in your life where you can enjoy more simplicity. Then make a plan of action of what you will implement and when. Commit to simplifying at least one area of your life in the next 3 days and then make it happen.

Chapter Fourteen

UPGRADES FOR A HEALTHIER LIFE

If you are not willing to learn, no one can help you. If you are determined to learn, no one can stop you.

— Zig Ziglar

An upgrade means simply to raise something to a higher standard, so when it comes to the foods you love to eat, an upgrade is choosing something that is of a higher quality. You could consider upgrades as a form of health insurance, similar to buying insurance to protect your personal belongings. Upgrading will help you protect your most important asset, your health.

We consider technological upgrades as necessary because they provide us with a better experience. We don't think twice about upgrading the software on our mobile device or computer. Using our frequent flier miles offers an inexpensive way to upgrade to a better seat providing a more comfortable experience when flying. There are many upgrades to choose from when it comes to eating healthier versions of your favorite foods.

I discovered this for myself as my passion and knowledge increased around investing in my health and wanting to eat better quality foods. I started to implement more upgrades whenever I found an alternative.

Everyday Product Upgrades

Let's consider upgrading some of the products you use often when making a home cooked meal.

Many of us use oil for cooking on a regular basis. I have switched from using olive oil for cooking with heat to using grape seed oil. We know that olive oil is high in heart-healthy antioxidants called polyphenols and monounsaturated fats, which can help lower "bad" LDL cholesterol and raise "good" HDL cholesterol levels, but if you are cooking over high heat, olive oil is not such a great option because it has a lower smoke point which is the point at which an oil literally begins to smoke (olive oil is between 365° and 420°F). When you heat olive oil to its smoke point, the beneficial compounds in the oil start to degrade, and potentially health-harming compounds form. Grape seed oil has a much higher smoke point of 485°F.

If you love to stir fry, try using Raw Coconut Aminos instead of regular soy sauce. It's a soy-free seasoning sauce which has only 113 mg of sodium per one teaspoon. It is substantially lower than other options including those that state it is lower in sodium. It's also an excellent alternative if you are trying to lower or maintain your blood pressure.

Another low sodium alternative is kelp granules. They can be used in place of regular salt either in cooking or as a condiment. They are also an excellent source of iodine for maintaining a healthy thyroid.

Stop Eating Genetically Modified Organisms (GMO's)

The definition of a GMO according to the Biology Department at the University of California San Diego is, "When a gene from one organism is purposely moved to improve or change another organism in a laboratory, the result is a genetically modified organism (GMO)." It is also sometimes called "transgenic" for transfer of genes. There are different ways of moving genes to produce desirable traits".

This is exactly what is happening to our food supply and the reason there is a movement to make GMO labelling on products in the U.S a legal requirement so consumers know what they are buying. It is very important to know what you are eating and avoid GMO foods as much as possible. Plan the time to shop mindfully and become informed about your choices to protect your most precious asset, your health. Don't be like me years ago, running around a supermarket so I could be finished sooner. Pay attention and your choices, and your health, will improve.

Reading Labels

Every time we make a purchase we are voting with our dollars. It's worth repeating that reading labels is so important and a great way to upgrade your choices. When you stop buying harmful products, it will not only benefit your health, but you send a strong message to the manufacturers who create products that are detrimental to your health. When there is a demand for a product, it will continue to be available for purchase. It will take a little time at first to discover the healthier choices available to you, but you are so worth it. I am such a lover of chocolate and I was delighted when I found an upgrade which has very few ingredients in it, and I can pronounce all the words. Switching to a healthier lifestyle might seem daunting at first, but as you now know, you can get started at any time of the year just by upgrading what you love, but you need to plan to make it happen.

Now you know you don't have to give up everything you love in order to lose weight and feel better. Just make a plan to implement some upgrades to get you started. It's a nice transition to eating what you enjoy, but in a much healthier way.

As you notice how much better you start to feel, you will naturally add more upgrades. It gets easier because you find pleasure in seeking out the best for yourself.

Chewing and Mindful Eating

All too often we tend to eat without being mindful of the experience and we end up missing the pure pleasure of meal times. We should be using all of our senses to enjoy the meal. Smell the aroma, see how bright and colorful your meal looks, hear the sizzle as it cooks, if appropriate feel it on your hands, but most importantly, taste your food and savor the experience.

Have you ever thought about how much you chew your food and the importance of chewing? In our fast-paced lives, eating can easily become something that is rushed. It is even done while multitasking, while driving or even on the run.

Planning enough time to eat your meals and chew your food thoroughly is a great way to upgrade how your body will feel during and after a meal. Digestion takes more energy than any other physiological function of the body, so if you are chewing each mouthful less than 30 times it could be one of the reasons you feel tired after a meal, because your body is working overtime to handle digestion. 30 times sounds a lot, but it isn't. I discovered this when I counted how many times I chew each mouthful and realized it was actually more than 30 times. Think of saliva as liquid gold. The more you chew and break down the food in your mouth, the more saliva you create. Digestive enzymes found in saliva begin to break the food down and help prepare for maximum absorption of vitamins and minerals. Saliva also assists in the digestion of carbohydrates and makes the food more alkaline, which creates less gas. One of the big problems in our society today is acidity in the body due to the Standard American Diet (S.A.D). Just like plants need a certain PH balance in the soil in order to thrive, we do too.

So many people chew their food very few times before swallowing, often without even realizing it. My clients are always thankful when I bring it to their attention. They had no clue about why this is so important.

Hands down, chewing each mouthful of food more times is a wonderful way to upgrade something you do many times a day. It will take practice at first and if you are eating with another person, ask them to help you slow down if you return to your fast pace. Plan to put your utensils down between each mouthful. It will definitely help to slow you down.

We usually have the next mouthful loaded up and in our mouths before we have even swallowed what we are already chewing. Try it out, but make it fun. Notice how differently you feel.

How to Improve Your Digestion

Digestion begins in the mouth where your tongue receives your food and it ends with a bowel movement. It has a big job to move food through a whole host of bodily functions. Digestive problems are a rapidly growing business in part, due to eating very acidic foods and a lack of proper digestion. A healthy gut is the foundation of good health. It takes between 2 to 6 hours for food to go through the stomach, so lying down too soon after a meal can be the cause of acid reflux. This simple change could be considered a fabulous upgrade if you suffer with acid reflux. When I exercise, I have to make sure that I have eaten 2 hours before, at a minimum, because when I bend over I get acid reflux since the food hasn't moved through my stomach.

Remember, a pill is a band-aid. You still have acid reflux if you haven't changed the foods or habits that are causing it. A little planning has huge rewards.

Review other areas of your life to discover where you may be experiencing digestive issues. Digestion isn't only about food. Are you consuming far too much information that you are struggling to digest and absorb? You know the saying "Don't bite off more than you can chew!"? Apart from foods that don't agree with you, what else is causing you discomfort?

Upgrades For a Healthier Life

Action Step

Upgrades are everywhere and become more obvious once we raise our awareness. What upgrades can you make in your life? I created an upgrade recommendation page that looks at two of my favorite areas to upgrade, chocolate and wine! It will help you look at these items in a way so you can see where you too can make an upgrade with your favorite treats. **www.DietFreeAndHealthy.com/bonus**

Chapter Fifteen

PRACTICAL TIPS FOR WHEREVER YOU ARE

Proper planning and preparation prevents
piss poor performance.
— A British Army adage

For many years when I was very active in the real estate business, my eating habits were less than desirable. I would often buy something from a gas station or have something I considered delicious with me like a bar of chocolate or cake, or even go for hours without eating. If I was still active in that industry, things would be very different for me because I would be prepared with an arsenal of nutritious foods to sustain me throughout the day.

I have avoided attending some events because I don't want to eat what is being served. I don't have any food allergies, but I do have a preference for eating quality food without pesticides and chemicals. It makes no sense for me to put myself in a situation where my digestion will be in agony for hours afterwards. So whenever possible, I either eat before going or I take some food with me. In the beginning, it felt a little awkward. I wasn't trying to draw attention to myself or imply that the food being served wasn't good enough for me, so it did feel a little tricky at times. I don't do this every single time, but I do use my judgment and common sense to determine if it's feasible given the circumstances.

Usually in less formal environments, it's perfectly fine. Somehow if someone is eating something different due to an allergy that seems acceptable, but not when they have a preference to passing up pesticides and chemicals.

Staying Healthy On the Go

If I am out and about for a few hours or more I will take a snack with me which is usually some left-overs that I put in a bowl, a handful of nuts, a piece of fruit or a smoothie. I just make sure I have something with me. This often seems a challenge for my clients in the beginning of working together, as they are not used to thinking of taking food with them or of using leftovers as a snack, but most of the time my leftovers are my snack and it is a great way to transition from consuming highly processed foods for snacks. I like to think of it as a mini-meal. Try it out for yourself. It will also save you time and money.

A Little Planning is Often All It Takes

Just like anything else in life you need a plan for making sure you have what you need with you to satisfy hunger and thirst during the day. Planning is a huge stepping stone to a healthier you. We plan for vacations, a wedding, a dinner party or a home improvement project. Your health and eating are no different, except this plan happens on a daily basis because this is a lifelong plan of action to keep you healthy and fit.

When I go on vacation or travel on business, I take as much of my own food with me because I know the quality of it. Remember, I used to eat out several nights a week if I could because I couldn't be bothered to cook. If I stay in a hotel, I call ahead and ask if there is a refrigerator in the room. I look online for a health food store closest to the hotel. I decide what I can pack to take with me and what I will buy when I get to my destination. I do eat out, but I limit it because I don't feel great afterwards. It's also a sure fire way to start putting back on the extra pounds in record time. The body knows what to do with real food. Starting out with a fairly modest plan while implementing these changes is a wonderful place to start.

Also, when traveling, I pack a few zip locks and a few containers and even a few sheets of paper towel. It might seem extreme, but I do it so automatically now and I love it because it means I stay feeling well and energized, instead of going back to feeling bloated and sluggish. In the beginning of traveling like this, I made a list of what I would take with me so that I didn't forget anything. You could start by creating a simple list that feels comfortable and not extreme to you. As you ease into doing this, you can start to upgrade the list by adding more to it. Some people create this kind of list for clothes and toiletries to pack when traveling. Taking some of your kitchen with you is not as difficult as it might seem. After all, we tend to take half our closets with us!

Think about this for a minute. A new mother with a baby or young child takes a bag full of all the things the baby will need while out of the house, such as diapers, wipes and nourishment. Why are we any different? We have needs while away from home, too. We know we will likely become hungry and thirsty, so making a plan to take food with you will go a long way towards creating a healthier life and keeping off the excess weight. It will become something that is automatic for you in no time.

Practical Tips for Wherever You Are

Action Step

Use the simple checklist found at **www.DietFreeAnd Healthy.com/ bonus** that you can place on your refrigerator to remind you how and what to pack when leaving the house. Using a tool like this will keep you focused on your health and help prevent situations where you could compromise your healthy choices.

Part Five

PASSION

Find something you're passionate about and keep tremendously interested in it.

—JULIA CHILD

Chapter Sixteen

LIGHTING UP YOUR FIRE

What are you currently passionate about in your life, really passionate? What lights you up whenever you think about it or talk about it and makes your heart sing? It doesn't have to be something monumental. In fact, it could be something simple, but it means a lot to you; it's somewhat effortless and it fills you with joy.

For me, helping people find freedom from their weight and health struggles as I did for myself really lights me up because it is transformational and sets people free. Donald Trump once said, "Your vocation should be like a vacation." This is exactly how I feel about my work. I love everything to do with helping others put the pieces of their health and happiness together. I read everything I can about health and wellness and spirituality because it not only helps my body and soul stay healthy as I age, but it lights me up deep within and that's the place I live from.

On the other hand, I have had jobs in the past that didn't really light my fire. I enjoy improving and simplifying systems, but once I had done what I could to make things run more efficiently I was not really fired up. It then became just a job. I am so fulfilled doing what I do now as a coach and mentor. I couldn't imagine doing anything else.

Always trying to lose weight and feeling hungry and deprived is one way to put out your fire. It's like the last log burning away before the fire eventually goes out. However, imagine feeling the strength and joy of a dancing fire about how you look and feel. Where you are not restricted or deprived and where you don't have to use discipline and structure. This has a whole different feel to it than the current ideas of what we are taught for losing weight without any focus on health.

What would it mean for you to be free of your food issues?

How would you define the freedom?

How would it make you feel?

Without passion, we have no results or poor results. We need passion for something in order to have the patience to stick with it and allow the process of learning, shifting, and transformation to unfold.

If you have ever learned to play a musical instrument or learned a foreign language, you may recall you had a passion for it initially, a desire which allowed you to be patient with learning and practicing, until you started to experience those exciting results of actually really playing the instrument or speaking a foreign language more fluently. It takes a little while before it becomes second nature. I have never felt passionate about going on a diet. However, I have become passionate about my health and the freedom I experience in my own life on a daily basis.

When you were a little girl chances are you really enjoyed dressing up your dolls. It was something that lit you up. It was so much fun to put them in different outfits and even mix and match. One Christmas, my parents gave my sister and I a box each of knitted custom clothes for our dolls that a friend had made. I think we had the same outfits in different colors. It was magical!

When was the last time you felt this excitement about getting yourself dressed every day? Do you feel like Negative Nancy or Passionate Pat going to your closet every day?

Feeling excited about going to my closet every day is something I now enjoy. I don't dread it in the summer months like I used to, when I couldn't layer up and hide what I didn't like about my figure.

Burn What Doesn't Fit Your Life

Just like the burning of bras as part of the Women's Liberation Movement back in the 60's and 70's, write down everything that doesn't serve you anymore and burn the piece of paper in the fireplace or outside as an act of liberation. This is very powerful. Include diets and even name them, emotions, relationships, thoughts, beliefs, etc. Just write down whatever you feel like letting go of and burn away. Everything is driven by the mind, so get rid of what doesn't serve you or light you up. Say goodbye to it for good. When we burn something, it is gone for good. What we focus on is what we manifest, so make room for what you really want more of in your life.

What puts out your fire? I find when I am using technology for too long it really dampens my spirit.

What feeds your fire? When I am out in nature, I feel grounded and supported and soak up the beauty which makes me feel alive.

Do you need praise to feel good in your life? I used to, but not anymore. Do you need acceptance to fully live your life? We all prefer to be accepted rather than ignored, but does it really matter?

Do you look to others to tell you what to do and how to do it? Is that why you have stayed stuck in patterns of dieting with your weight going up and down like a yo-yo? If we had the unfortunate experience of being stuck in an elevator, we would want to be rescued as quickly as possible. Unfortunately, we stay stuck in old beliefs and traditions for years that keep our internal flame turned down low.

Let's Get Your Fire Burning Brightly

Do you remember the fire in your belly for wanting to pass a test you had been studying for? Any kind of test, such as a driving test, real estate, hairdressing, etc. or getting your degree or a certification in your chosen profession? Passing the test would add value to your life in some way and you had a passion for it.

Well, I have a proposition for you. I encourage you to get just as excited about your blood work test results. Yes, your blood work test results! Many doctors don't mail out a copy of patient blood work, my primary doctor included. I have to ask for a copy. Sometimes, even when my numbers have been out of range, I only found out because I requested a copy and I reviewed the information and researched natural ways to course correct. Things don't usually improve by themselves. We study for a test, so let's study what's going on with your body. Blood work reveals a lot about what is going on in your body and I believe it is crucial to be proactive in keeping track of how you are doing. Isn't this the ultimate test to pass in life, enjoying long-term health? I have become very passionate about my blood work results. I love seeing a glowing review, but sometimes I still need to make improvements so that I get an even better result. I am passionate about keeping everything in good order because as we age, the domino effect can quickly start to happen. Before you know it, there's another problem and another problem.

Vitamin D "The Sunshine Vitamin"

I am not a fan of humidity, but I do love to feel the sun on my skin. I love it when the weather is warm enough to expose my feet so they can breathe again after being in boots all winter. I am a big proponent of doing things the natural way whenever possible and that includes getting my vitamin D from the sun to avoid ongoing supplementation. However, there seems to be conflicting information when it comes to supplementing with vitamin D. In addition, we have been told to limit our time in the sun and to use sun screen. But, the most natural way to build up your vitamin D level is by being in the sun. The body can only store vitamin D from the sun and not supplementation.

I make a conscious effort to go outside as often as possible when it's warm enough. I'll stay outside for just 10 to 15 minutes per day, which helps to prevent burning. I expose my arms, shoulders and legs. Even though this is my first choice, I have not always been successful with raising my levels to an adequate level, so on occasion I do supplement with a liquid form of vitamin D. Low levels of vitamin D is detrimental to our health, so I take it very seriously and I recommend that you do, too.

We spend so much time indoors these days preventing us from getting adequate sunshine, but it also disconnects us from being in nature and enjoying all the beauty of flowers, aromas, the sounds of the birds, wind and the animals going about their day. When we think of connecting with nature in this way, we will want to blend with it and develop an attitude that getting enough sunlight for vitamin D is necessary and not a "health chore" but something you feel passionate about doing.

Vitamin B12 "The Energy Vitamin"

The older you get the more likely you are to have a vitamin B12 deficiency. Vitamin B12, known as the energy vitamin, impacts a number of very important systems in your body, everything from your DNA to how happy you feel. If you are feeling like your fire has gone out, it is worth having your B12 level checked. The more intimate you become with the needs of your body and what it is communicating to you, you will become your own health detective and know when something is off because you will be familiar with the feelings. I don't recommend supplements often, but sometimes they are necessary for a specific period of time. Just like processed food, be sure to read the ingredient label and buy the best quality possible.

Lighting Up Your Fire

Action Step

Ask your doctor for a copy of your last two blood work test results if you don't already have them. Review the information and start monitoring how you are doing, not because you feel it's something you should do, but because it lights you up to know how well you are doing. Getting good results is something to get excited about, especially by doing it the natural way and not by taking harmful medications. Ask for a copy every time going forward and keep track of how you are doing. I've put together a list of some of the basic tests you should look at to help you become more proactive in making the best decisions possible for your health. You can see it at: **www.DietFreeAndHealthy.com/bonus**

Chapter Seventeen

AWARENESS WITHOUT ATTACHMENT

Awareness

Across the landscape, I stand and stare,

And I feel what it's like to be aware.

Aware of everything inside and out.

And I understand what life is about.

I stay aware of what I think,

I'm aware of what I eat and drink.

I'm aware of my feelings, large and small.

I'm aware when I falter, and when I stand tall.

When I'm aware, I am free.

That's when I'm the I AM me!

I flow through life with wonderous ease,

Doing anything that I please!

Geri Jones – www.PomesByJones.com

The first self-help book I read back in the 80's was called *You Can Heal Your Life* by Louise Hay. I started to awaken and found the subject matter very interesting. I took classes in learning about energy fields, chakras and even how food can negatively or positively affect our own energy field. I took some shamanic healing classes. I read a lot more books. I was fascinated by discovering more about who I am, and why I am here. I took workshops regarding self-improvement. The learning has escalated because of my passion for looking and feeling great. I continue to learn and peel the layers of the onion away in my life, letting go of what doesn't serve my highest good and living from a place of purpose and passion.

When I believe in something or someone, I used to hang on their every word and practically perform what they said to the letter. But, sometimes it just didn't seem to fit me. Something seemed off. I realized I should take what feels right to me and leave the rest because it is someone else's interpretation of how things should be. This really opened me up to more learning and receiving instead of pigeon holing myself into one belief or way of doing things.

Awareness Is a Gift for Change

A friend of mine once told me that she read an interesting book about chakras. She went on to say that the author was challenging the fact that they even exist. Even though I am open to a good discussion about different sides of a topic, I told her that I believe they do exist and I said that everyone has an opinion, but we should each listen to what resonates with us. She liked my response and told me that I have "awareness without attachment". These words have stuck with me ever since. No one, including myself, had ever summed up my observation and decision before of "taking what feels right and leaving the rest."

Staying Open to All Possibilities

Have you ever followed a teaching or belief about what you should do to look and feel better, but didn't end up looking or feeling better? Yes, me too!

I am aware of many different approaches to health and wellness, but I am not attached to any one belief system where I follow it to the letter. My hope for you is that you pay attention to what resonates with you, rather than being a sheep and following the herd. I enjoy some things from one school of thought and some from others. Please don't just hand your power over to someone else because they say it is so. Listen to your own gut feeling about whether it makes sense for you.

I am a big fan of common sense, and if it doesn't make sense to me, I don't do it. The whole purpose of this book is not to tell you what to do, but rather to open you up and awaken you to a new way that empowers you.

Vegan or Vegetarian

Many people who become vegetarians often do so at a young age because of how they feel emotionally about animals. I totally understand. So many animals raised in factory farms for human consumption live in such awful conditions and in fear. We ingest the energy of these frightened animals. I am very opposed to any kind of cruelty and suffering. The decision to be vegan or vegetarian may have been the right one for them at the time; however, it might not be such a good choice for their body as they get older because the needs of the body do change. There is an alternative choice to being vegan or vegetarian for animal cruelty reasons. There is a video about Deep Roots Meat, a humane farm that was showcased in the documentary *Food, Inc.* **www.DietFreeAnd Healthy.com/deep-roots-meat**, where some vegetarians are now buying meat.

I have never personally been a huge meat eater, but as I have developed more awareness about listening to the needs of my body, I do notice that I do well on a small amount of animal protein. I make sure that what I am eating had a pleasant happy life.

In fact, when I was a kid I had a hard time swallowing meat. I would chew and chew, but it never seemed to break down in my mouth so I could swallow it, especially if it was red meat. My auntie was a dinner lady at my infant and junior school, and she would bring around a piece of paper towel so that I could put the contents from my mouth in it. At home, I would put small pieces of the meat I couldn't swallow around the edge of my plate and it became a bit of a family joke.

Since learning about the 4 different blood types O, A, B and AB, during my holistic health training, I was curious to find out my own blood type. I am A Positive and this blood type, according to Dr. Peter J. D'Adamo, the creator of *The Blood Type Diet*, is best suited to a classic, vegan or vegetarian diet. I found this fascinating. Perhaps my body was telling me I didn't need meat by not being able to swallow it. Interesting! My husband's blood type on the other hand is O Positive and he does feel the need to eat meat. O blood types actually have strong enzymes to digest it.

I also find the other facts about the blood type approach to diet and health fascinating, such as O types are most susceptible to wheat and corn allergies, but I am not attached to following it to the letter. I do enjoy having the awareness that it exists as a resource for looking at the whole picture of health and our unique dietary needs. I believe it is good to have a repertoire of knowledge, but to use it wisely in the way that fits us best.

Raw Food

Some people think that raw is the way to go regardless of the season. Traditional Chinese Medicine advocates not eating raw food in the cold dead of winter. This ancient tradition believes that food should be slowly cooked during the cold winter months, which makes sense to me. We need foods that warm the body. Not foods that cool the body and potentially weaken it. The opposite is true in the hot weather. We need cooling foods, but many eat a lot of food that is hot from cooking it on the grill.

I went to one of the finest raw food restaurants in NYC a few years ago. The food is absolutely top notch. The presentation is wonderful and everything is very fresh. I tried a few different dishes with my friend Maria, one of which was a fantastic "burger" made with portobello mushroom and manna bread. On the train ride home it felt like I had cement stuck in my gut. I was so uncomfortable. I felt exhausted and I didn't feel well at all. My digestion was on overload. The next day, I thankfully had my regular acupuncture appointment and within no time at all the energy was moving again. My system doesn't do well on a lot of raw food, especially if it is not predigested by being blended or juiced. Have you experienced feeling tired and uncomfortable after eating too much raw food? If so, this could be the reason. Remember, we are all unique. Food and philosophy is never one-size fits all. Listen to your body. It will let you know if it is happy or unhappy with you.

Juicing/Detoxing

There are certainly die hard juicers out there, but I'm not one of them and certainly not for extended periods of time. I do believe in juicing and I approach it as part of investing in my health. Not something that is done 100% for days on end without any other food. The fiber is removed when the juice is extracted from the pulp, so for someone who isn't eating vegetables in some other form they are missing out on the fiber. Including blends in a detox made in a blender such as a Vitamix can take care of this because the vegetables are completely intact.

I like to detox twice a year, usually in the spring when the weather is just getting warm enough and nature is coming back to life, and also in late summer just before the fall. I have a green drink to start off the day and then the other 5 drinks are blends made in the Vitamix. I do this for 3 to 5 days each time. Some promote juicing/detoxing several times a year. I don't recommend this, especially if it doesn't match the rhythm of nature. In the dead of winter, nature is sleeping. Nothing is really active and a detox is very forceful on the body because it promotes the removal of toxins. I believe that cleaning out toxins from the body is a wonderful thing when following the rhythm of nature. I am usually hungrier in the winter months and a detox would not make me feel happy and satisfied.

I still have one juice a day from time to time during the winter, but I also eat plenty of warm slow cooked delicious meals. I like the way I feel when I have a vegetable juice, so I do like to include it for this reason. When I make a juice for clients that I see in person, they look and feel different within 15 minutes. They can hardly believe how it improves how they feel, which gives them motivation for doing it themselves.

Marathon runners get their body ready for the big race months ahead of time. They don't just show up unfit and hope for the best. Take time to get your body in better health before going all out on a detox marathon.

Live Your Life by Design and Not by Default

- What is your body saying to you?

- Does it feel happy when you eat meat?

- Does it crave meat when you don't eat it?

- Do you detox and crave the whole time you are on the detox?

- Do you welcome a detox as a natural extension of your approach to overall health?

I advocate that we each listen to the needs of our body instead of following a structured plan or belief system. You be the ultimate judge and jury for your body and life.

Find the passion in everything you do. If something makes you miserable, don't do it. If you don't feel happy on a detox, don't do one just because it seems like a good idea. When you are ready, you will fully embrace it in mind, body and spirit and be delighted with your decision to give yourself this healthy gift.

Awareness Without Attachment

Action Step

I created a video to help you identify the areas in your life where you are doing things you don't enjoy. You can use this information to transition to making choices for your health that will make you passionate about creating healthier choices for yourself. To watch the video, go to:

www.DietFreeAndHealthy.com/bonus

Chapter Eighteen

CELEBRATE EVERYTHING

How often do we forget to sit back and praise ourselves for what we have accomplished? I have a tendency to feel thankful for when I have accomplished something, but I don't often take the time to really stop and bask in it by taking a breather until I move onto the next thing.

Would you have ever considered celebrating cleaning up your sock drawer prior to reading about how clutter can negatively affect your health? Probably not, because who would celebrate doing that? Celebrate every single thing that contributes to living a healthier and happier life. I mean EVERYTHING!

Please develop the art of celebrating everything, even something that you consider small. One of my clients who never read labels said to me she only read two labels when she went to buy her groceries after we spoke about it. I told her that was great news because it's two more than she read before. She didn't see it as something to celebrate because it didn't seem big enough. We all want to feel like we are doing good things in the world, but let's acknowledge the good we are doing for ourselves.

Going from no water a day to two glasses a day is cause for celebration. Drinking one less cup of coffee a day is cause for celebration. Eating out one less time per week is cause for celebration.

We celebrate special days and events in other people's lives by giving them gifts, so why not celebrate everything we do for ourselves as we shower ourselves with daily gifts. It doesn't matter if it's big or small. A gift is still a gift and it's the thought that counts. Start counting the gifts you can give to yourself regularly.

Adore yourself. Be compassionate with yourself and express gratitude every day.

Here's to celebrating you and bringing more meaning to your life.

Cheers!

Celebrate Everything

Action Step

Use the celebration fund examples at **www.DietFreeAnd Healthy.com/bonus** to discover how you can continue celebrating the new healthy choices you are making.

CONCLUSION

My heart is so full of excitement that you have chosen to embrace the GIFT of health and happiness to yourself and turn your focus away from the drama of diets and harmful medications that only manage and mask a problem, instead of healing it.

Remember that change is possible when you make yourself a *Priority*. When you stop *Pretending* about your reality. When you shift your *Perception* about how you see things. When you have a *Plan* and when you have *Passion*.

This is not a sprint to the finish line, so go with a pace you are comfortable with. I was where you are. I had weight issues on and off for years. The beautiful thing now is that I no longer have an issue. Not because my weight doesn't ever fluctuate, but because I don't consider it an issue. I do not have any attachment or judgment either way. Being healthy and kind to myself is what matters the most to me.

Keep telling yourself you are worthy of a body and life you love, take baby steps, celebrate everything you accomplish and keep looking back to see just how far you have come!

To Your Health and Happiness,

— Ellie

ACKNOWLEDGEMENTS

My husband and best friend Ralph Savoy Jr., for supporting me in everything I do and loving me unconditionally.

My mother, Joyce Whitmore, who taught me many practical things in my life such as how to get on with things even when you don't feel like doing them, not to complain and how to be strong.

My dad, Tony Whitmore, "the King of the Sky" who taught me compassion, kindness, a strong work ethic and so much more. Hardly a day goes by without some reference to a lesson he shared with me throughout my life. He was a natural philosopher.

My friend Betty Renner, who has supported me in all my endeavors and is a big fan of me writing my first book and getting my message to more people.

My friend Stella Levak, for providing a new set of eyes for reading this book and offering refinements.

My friend and acupuncturist Thérèse Balagna, who has supported me in my personal growth and development, and healing over many years.

My business partner Rory Carruthers, who contributed so much to making this book a reality.

My editor, Carly Carruthers, who provided so much more than checking grammar and punctuation.

My wonderful clients, who I learn so much from everyday.

Everyone who has enriched my life, you know who you are.

REFERENCES

Here are a few resources that have been helpful for me and my clients. If you did not get a chance to explore, watch, or purchase these resources while reading the book, here is a list of all of the resources mentioned within the chapters of *Stop Dieting Start Living.*

Websites:

- Diet Free and Healthy - "The Life You Deserve" My website provides more information about the diet free and healthy experience. Get access to blog entries, interviews, and additional videos, plus much more to help you stay on the path of healthy living!
  www.DietFreeAndHealthy.com

- Pomes by Jones - Inspirational poems to fuel your soul and keep you motivated. Poems can even be personalized!
  www.PomesByJones.com

- Local Harvest - "Real food, Real Farmers, Real Community" A great place to find local farms, farmers markets, CSAs, and agricultural events in your area. **www.LocalHarvest.org**

- Mercola - "Take Control of Your Health" A natural health website with current health news and quality products. **www.Mercola.com**

Videos:

- *Death by Sugar* - Video showing how sugar negatively affects our overall health. **www.DietFreeAnd Healthy.com/death-by-sugar**

- *Forks Over Knives* - Documentary about how food can be used as medicine. **www.DietFreeAndHealthy.com/forks-over-knives**

- *Deep Roots Meat* - "Featured in the documentary film "Food Inc.", Troy's ranch is a model for what land stewardship and humane treatment of farm animals ought to be." **www.DietFreeAnd Healthy.com/deep-roots-meat**

Books:

- *Raw Food Made Easy for 1 to 2 People* by Jennifer Cornbleet- "Well-known Bay Area cooking instructor, Jennifer Cornbleet, shares her favorite no-cook recipes in quantities ideal for one or two people. With essential time-saving tips and techniques, plus with Jennifer's clear instructions, you don't have to toil in the kitchen in order to enjoy nutritious, delicious raw food." **www.DietFree AndHealthy.com/raw-food-made-easy**

- *You Can Heal Your Life* by Louise Hay- "Louise L. Hay, bestselling author, is an internationally known leader in the self-help field. Her key message is: 'If we are willing to do the mental work, almost anything can be healed.' The author has a great deal of experience and firsthand information to share about healing, including how she cured herself after being diagnosed with cancer." **www.DietFreeAndHealthy.com/you-can-heal-your-life**

About the Author

ELLIE SAVOY is a #1 International Bestselling Author and a Holistic Health Coach. She is also the founder of Diet Free and Healthy, the revolutionary health and weight loss system for women.

Born and raised in England, Ellie married young and was divorced by 30. She didn't know who she was or what she wanted from life. She had always put everyone and everything ahead of herself. Ellie came to the US to visit and experience more of what the world had to offer. She had no intention of staying, but as fate would have it she met the man who would become her husband. Feeling homesick though Ellie really wanted to jump into a career.

She quickly gravitated to the Real Estate field, moving up the ranks quickly and winning awards for her work. In 2002 Ellie opened her own Real Estate firm and became the most leading edge and forward thinking brokerage in her area. She single handedly pioneered the use of MLS services on her website to show all homes available for sale in the area, something that all agents now do. Clients loved Ellie's passion and dedication to helping them find the right home for them. But it wasn't all roses and daffodils.

The cost of a grueling schedule mixed with an unending desire to keep her real estate firm successful took its toll on Ellie's health. She was exhausted and overweight. She would literally jog through the grocery store throwing food in her cart haphazardly, and without thought of what was in the food, because she didn't have the time to be in the store. Something had to give and she suffered because of these choices.

After the sudden death of both of her parents in a short period of time, Ellie began to re-evaluate her priorities in life. Her real journey began in the summer of 2011 when she was diagnosed with uterine fibroids.

She was given four options, three involved surgery and the forth was to do nothing. The idea of surgery was unappealing and in typical Ellie fashion, doing nothing was not an option. This shocking moment made Ellie realize the errors of her ways. She started a journey of self healing, and ended up stumbling upon the real secret to weight loss.

Since then Ellie has dedicated her life to helping women all over the world improve their health and let go of excess weight without resorting to dieting or harmful weight loss pills. Ellie's message that women don't have to suffer in silence, live with pain or resort to harmful dieting practices to lose weight has resonated with women since day one.

Ellie's work is the culmination of not only her experiences and accomplishments, but of the success of her clients as well. To meet Ellie and find out more about how you can take your health and weight loss goals to the next level without dieting visit:

www.DietFreeAndHealthy.com